Table of Contents

Puzzle #1:   Drug Action: Absorption

Puzzle #2:   Drug Action: Distribution

Puzzle #3:   Drug Action: Metabolism

Puzzle #4:   Drug Action: Excretion

Puzzle #5:   Drug Action: Accumulation & Disease & Age

Puzzle #6:   Principles of Medication Administration

Puzzle #7:   Administration of Oral Medications

Puzzle #8:   Administration of Rectal Drugs

Puzzle #9:   Administration of Nasal Medications

Puzzle #10:   Administration of Inhalants

Puzzle #11:   Administration of Ophthalmic Medications

Puzzle #12:   Administration of Otic Medications

Puzzle #13:   Administration of Topical Agents

Puzzle #14:   Administration of Vaginal Medications

Puzzle #15:   Administration of Parenteral Medications

Puzzle #16:   Local Anesthetics

Puzzle #17:   Nonnarcotic Analgesics and Antipyretics

Puzzle #18:   Narcotic Analgesics

Puzzle #19:   Narcotic Antagonists

Puzzle #20:   Sedatives and Hypnotics

Puzzle #21:   Anticonvulsants

Puzzle #22:   Muscle Relaxants

Puzzle #23:   Antipsychotic Agents I

Puzzle #24:   Antipsychotic Agents II

Puzzle #25:   Antipsychotic Agents III

Puzzle #26:   Direct-Acting Adrenergics

Puzzle #27:   Adrenergic Blocking Agents

Puzzle #28:   Cholinergics

Puzzle #29:   Anticholinergics

Puzzle #30:   Antiparkinson Agents

Puzzle #31:   Hypothalamus and Pituitary Gland

Puzzle #32:   Thyroid, Parathyroid and Adrenal Glands

Puzzle #33:   Pancreas, Ovaries, Testes and Pineal Gland

Puzzle #34:   Thymus, GI tract, Placenta, Kidneys, Heart, Adipose Tissue, Eicosanoids, and Growth Factors

Puzzle #35:   Antidiabetic Agents

Puzzle #36:   Pituitary Hormones

Puzzle #37:   Corticosteroids

Puzzle #38:   Thyroid Hormones

Puzzle #39:   Thyroid Antagonists

Puzzle #40:   Women's Health Agents

Puzzle #41:   Men's Health Agents

Puzzle #42:   Oxytocics

Puzzle #43:   Mydriatics and Cycloplegics

Puzzle #44:   Miotics

Puzzle #45:   Cardiac Glycosides

Puzzle #46:   Antiarrhythmic Drugs

Puzzle #47:   Antianginal Drugs

Puzzle #48:   Peripheral Vasodilators and Antidysrhythmics I

Puzzle #49:   Antidysrhythmics II

Puzzle #50:   Beta Blockers

Puzzle #51:   Cardiac Stimulants

Puzzle #52:   Anticoagulants

Puzzle #53:   Thrombolytic Drugs

Puzzle #54:   Antilipemic Agents

Puzzle #55:   Antihypertensives I

Puzzle #56:   Antihypertensives II

Drug Action: Absorption

Dr. Evelyn J. Biluk

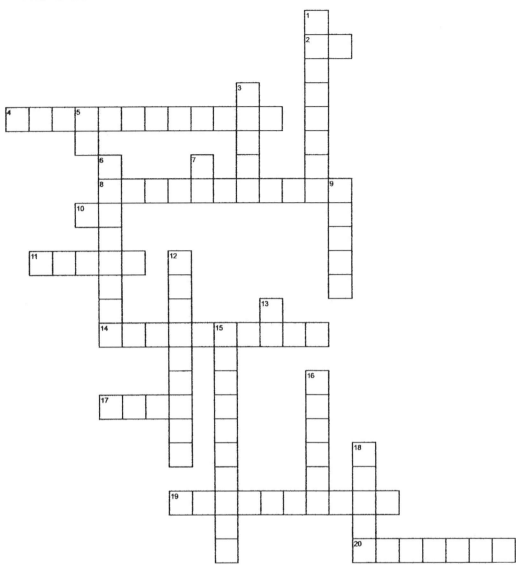

Drug Action: Absorption
Dr. Evelyn J. Biluk

Across

2.   Intravenous (_____) route is the most rapid absorption

4.   _____ can also delay drug absorption and potentially cause toxicity

8.   _____ route; Absorption is slow and confined to the injected area (e.g., PPD)

10.   Intramuscular (_____) route; Absorption is relatively fast

11.   _____ will delay absorption of drugs by the IM and SC routes

14.   _____ is the time it takes for a drug to enter the body until entrance into the blood

17.   _____ route; Rate and degree of absorption depends on GI motility, presence of food in stomach, gastric pH and the use of other drugs

19.   _____ circulation can also delay absorption of drugs by the IM and SC routes

20.   The _____ empties more slowly with food resulting in a delay of oral drug absorption

Down

1.   _____ can cause drugs not to be absorbed

3.   The _____ of administration affects the rate and amount of absorption

5.   Subcutaneous (_____) route; Absorption is also relatively fast

6.   Lipid solubility affects the absorption of drugs as it passes through the _____

7.   Intra-arterial (_____) is also one of two most rapid absorption routes

9.   _____ solubility affects the rate and amount of absorption

12.   The speed of absorption by the IM and SC route depends on the condition of _____

13.   Gastrointestinal (_____) motility affects the rate and amount of absorption

15.   A route of administration; Generally a rapid route

16.   _____ form affects the rate and amount of absorption

18.   Most oral drugs are best absorbed if given before or between _____

Drug Action: Absorption

Dr. Evelyn J. Biluk

Word bank

ABSORPTION   BLOODFLOW   CONSTIPATION   DIARRHEA   DOSAGE   GI   GIMUCOSA   IA   IM

INTRADERMAL   IV   LIPID   MEALS   ORAL   PARENTERAL   PERIPHERAL   ROUTE   SC   SHOCK

STOMACH

Drug Action: Absorption

Dr. Evelyn J. Biluk

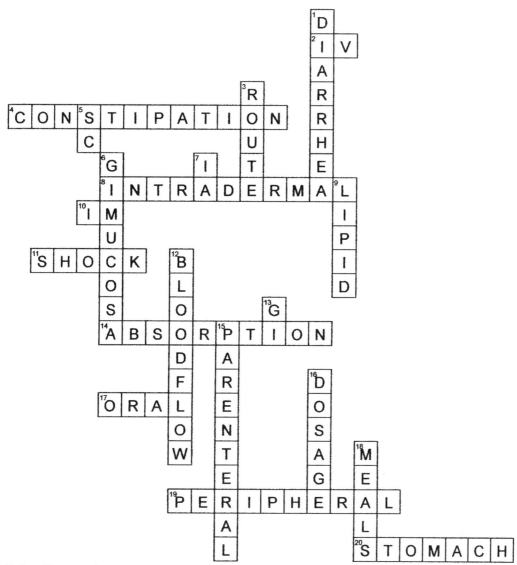

EclipseCrossword.com

Drug Action: Distribution

Dr. Evelyn J. Biluk

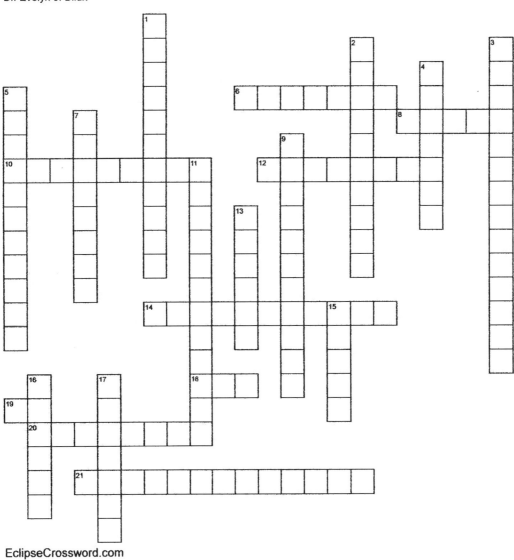

Drug Action: Distribution

Dr. Evelyn J. Biluk

Across

6.   _____ plays a role in drug distribution because blood flows through fat slowly thereby increasing the time before the drug is released

8.   Distribution of drugs using the blood can take as long as several _____ depending on blood flow and cardiac output

10.   _____ barrier shields the fetus from the possibility of drug effects

12.   An agonist drug will connect itself to a receptor and cause a pharmacological _____

14.   Once in the _____, drugs are distributed throughout the human body

18.   Aka blood brain barrier; Barrier to drug distribution

19.   An antagonist drug will attempt to attach itself to a receptor but because attachment is uneven, there is _____ pharmacological response

20.   _____ can cross the placental barrier as well as drugs and alcohol

21.   Clients with _____ or liver disease who have reduced plasma proteins could receive a heightened drug effect

Down

1.   BBB helps preserve _____ in the brain

2.   Drugs can also have an _____ effect; Opposite of agonist

3.   Medications connect with _____ in the vascular system

4.   Receptors for drugs can be made out of _____ or nucleic acids usually

5.   _____ at the receptor site can occur when more than one drug tries to occupy it

7.   A cell area where the drug attaches and a response occurs

9.   Clients with _____ may need a smaller dose of a drug

11.   To pass through the BBB, a drug must be _____ and loosely attached to plasma proteins

13.   Other substances such as _____ can be receptors for drugs on cells

15.   Clients with _____ may need an increased dose of a drug

16.   Strong attachments between a medication and plasma proteins may result in a _____ period of drug action

17.   Drugs can have an _____ effect

Drug Action: Distribution

Dr. Evelyn J. Biluk

Word bank

AGONIST   ANTAGONIST   BBB   BLOODSTREAM   COMPETITION   DEHYDRATION   EDEMA

HOMEOSTASIS   HOURS   KIDNEYDISEASE   LIPIDS   LIPIDSOLUBLE   LONGER   NICOTINE   NO

OBESITY   PLACENTAL   PLASMAPROTEINS   PROTEIN   RECEPTOR   RESPONSE

Drug Action: Distribution

Dr. Evelyn J. Biluk

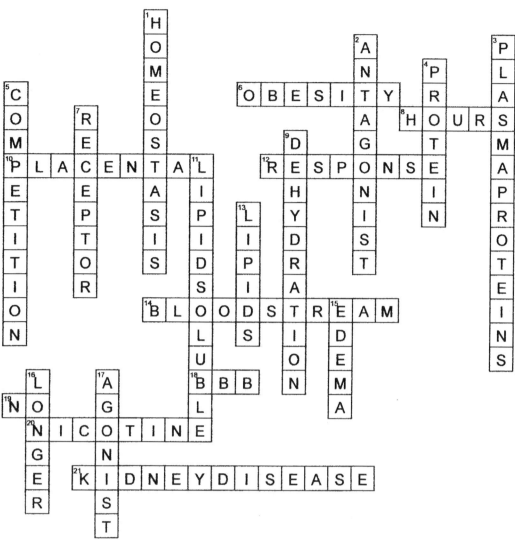

EclipseCrossword.com

Drug Action: Metabolism

Dr. Evelyn J. Biluk

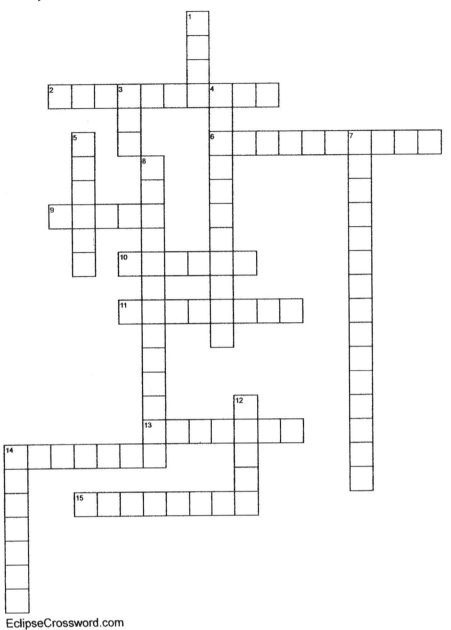

EclipseCrossword.com

Drug Action: Metabolism

Dr. Evelyn J. Biluk

Across

2. Sequence of chemical events that can change a drug after entering the human body

6. Liver enzymes involved in metabolism rely on adequate amounts of _____ (building blocks of proteins)

9. Principal organ involved in drug metabolism

10. Oral meds go to the liver via the _____ circulation

11. Oral meds go to the liver first and then end up in _____ circulation

13. _____ also have reduced ability to metabolize some drugs

14. _____ have reduced ability to metabolize some drugs

15. Liver enzymes involved in metabolism rely on adequate amounts of _____ (e.g., A, D, E, K, B, C)

Down

1. _____ medications go directly to the liver

3. The _____ of an individual influences the metabolism of drugs

4. Many medications become entirely _____ by the liver their first time thru

5. Liver enzymes involved in metabolism rely on adequate amounts of _____ (fats)

7. Insufficient amounts of adrenal _____ can reduce the metabolism of drugs in the liver

8. Liver enzymes involved in metabolism rely on adequate amounts of _____ (sugars)

12. _____ are metabolized in the liver

14. Insufficient amounts of this pancreatic hormone can reduce the metabolism of drugs in the liver

Drug Action: Metabolism

Dr. Evelyn J. Biluk

Word bank

AGE   AMINOACIDS   CARBOHYDRATES   CORTICOSTEROIDS   DRUGS   ELDERLY   INACTIVATED

INFANTS   INSULIN   LIPIDS   LIVER   METABOLISM   ORAL   PORTAL   SYSTEMIC   VITAMINS

Drug Action: Metabolism

Dr. Evelyn J. Biluk

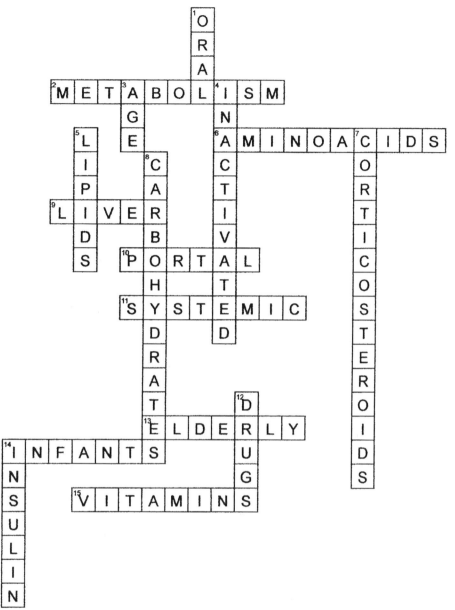

Drug Action: Excretion

Dr. Evelyn J. Biluk

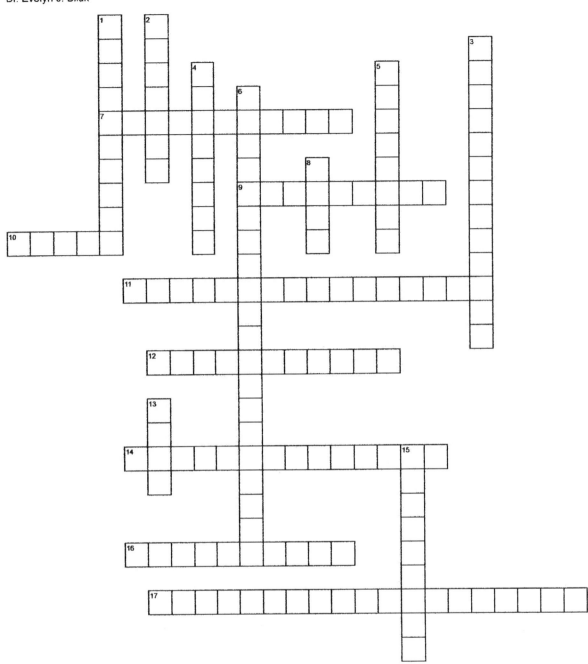

Drug Action: Excretion
Dr. Evelyn J. Biluk

Across

7. Drugs can be excreted by _____ (integumentary system); Apocrine and eccrine are subtypes

9. Process in which drugs are eliminated from the human body

10. Drugs can be excreted by _____ (respiratory system)

11. Renal excretion is carried out by _____ at the distal convoluted tubule primarily

12. Drugs can affect the _____ of other drugs

14. Drugs can be excreted by _____ (integumentary system); *Salivary, mandibular and sublingual are subtypes*

16. _____ is administered with penicillin to increase the effects of penicillin

17. _____ allows drug metabolites in the urine to re-enter the bloodstream

Down

1. Drugs can be excreted by _____ (digestive system)

2. Drugs can excreted by the _____ (urinary system); Most important drug excretion route

3. Drugs can be excreted by _____ (integumentary system)

4. _____ increase the elimination of aspirin

5. The time required for the total amount of a drug to decrease by 50 percent

6. Renal excretion is carried out by _____ at Bowman's capsule

8. When peak blood levels of a drug are reached, excretion increases and then blood levels of the drug begin to _____

13. When _____ blood levels of a drug are reached, excretion becomes greater than absorption

15. Tubular reabsorption _____ the quantity of drug excreted in the urine

Drug Action: Excretion

Dr. Evelyn J. Biluk

Word bank

ANTACIDS   DECREASES   DROP   ELIMINATION   EXCRETION   GLOMERULARFILTRATION   HALFLIFE

INTESTINES   KIDNEYS   LUNGS   MAMMARYGLANDS   PEAK   PROBENECID   SALIVARYGLANDS

SWEATGLANDS   TUBULARREABSORPTION   TUBULARSECRETION

Drug Action: Excretion

Dr. Evelyn J. Biluk

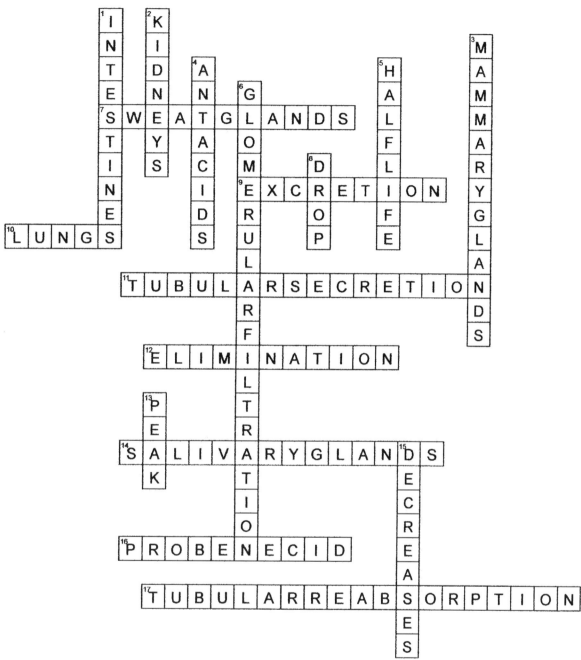

Drug Action: Accumulation & Disease & Age

Dr. Evelyn J. Biluk

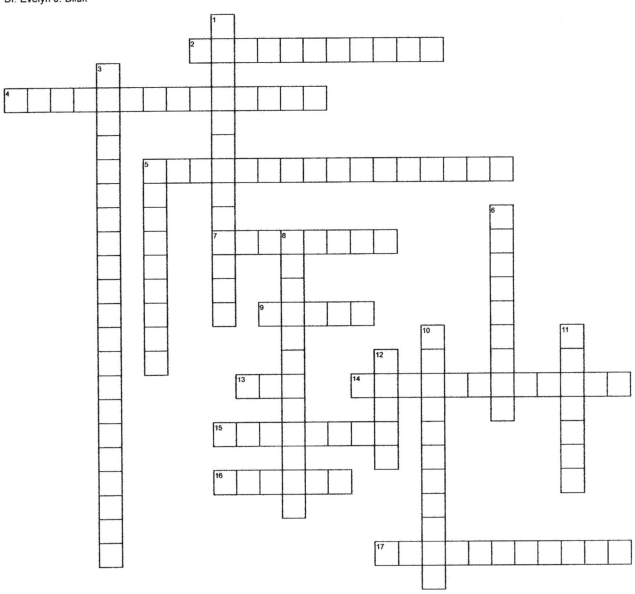

Drug Action: Accumulation & Disease & Age
Dr. Evelyn J. Biluk

Across

2. _____ can be given to raise the therapeutic level quickly before drug elimination

4. _____ (heart/blood vessels) disease can affect drug response

5. _____ (GI) disease can affect drug response

7. _____ happens when a drug is eliminated more slowly than it is absorbed

9. When _____ (urinary system) function remains unchanged, therapeutic levels can be maintained

13. AKA over the counter drugs

14. _____ can affect drug response (2 words)

15. Diseases can lead to _____ drug responses

16. _____ (urinary system) disease can affect drug response

17. Once the therapeutic level is achieved, a smaller daily _____ dose of a drug is given to maintain therapeutic levels

Down

1. Toxicity causes excessive drug _____

3. Units of pediatric drug dosages

5. A careful drug history needs to be obtained from an elderly client before determining _____ drug dosage

6. _____ drug dosages are based on body weight

8. Potential drug _____ with OTC drugs must be determined for geriatric clients

10. It is important for a drug to reach and maintain _____ levels

11. Loading doses are given in several _____ doses

12. Therapeutic levels can be maintained when _____ (digestive system) function remains unchanged

Drug Action: Accumulation & Disease & Age

Dr. Evelyn J. Biluk

Word bank

CARDIOVASCULAR   CONCENTRATION   GASTROINTESTINAL   GERIATRIC   INTERACTIONS   KIDNEY   LIVER   LIVERDISEASE   LOADINGDOSE   MAINTENANCE   MILLIGRAMSPERKILOGRAM   OTC   PEDIATRIC   RENAL   SMALLER   THERAPEUTIC   TOXICITY   VARIABLE

Drug Action: Accumulation & Disease & Age

Dr. Evelyn J. Biluk

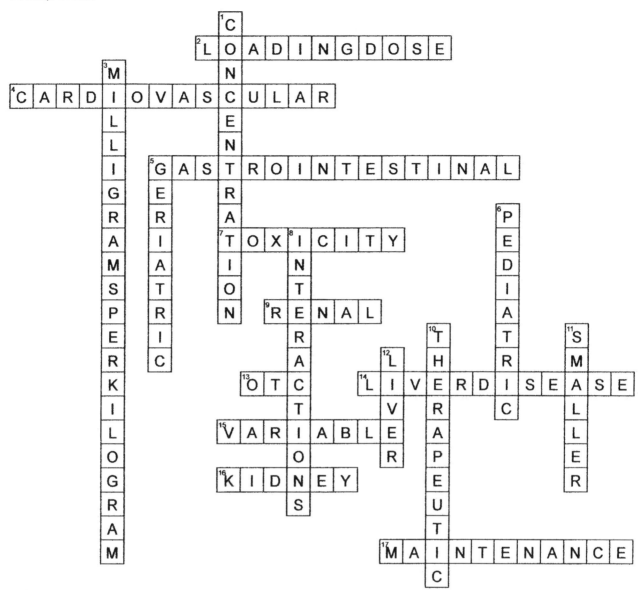

EclipseCrossword.com

Principles of Medication Administration

Dr. Evelyn J. Biluk

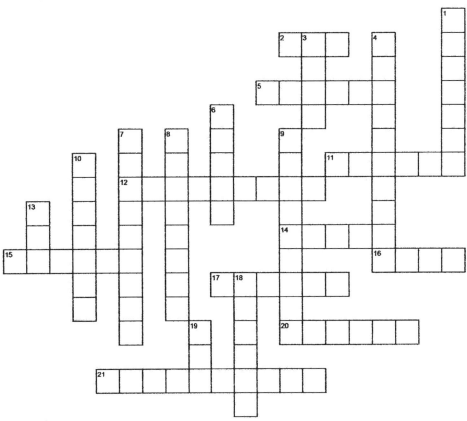

Principles of Medication Administration

Dr. Evelyn J. Biluk

Across

2. Confirm client's ID by checking at least _____ of the three possible mechanism for identification

5. Calculate _____ accurately

11. Give medication within _____ minutes of prescribed time

12. Observe _____ precautions

14. Compare label _____ times with the medication to decrease error risk

15. _____ client of medication, any procedure, technique, purpose and client teaching if applicable

16. Research _____ compatibilities, action, purpose, contraindications, side effects and appropriate routes

17. Report any _____ immediately and complete appropriate documentation

20. Review MAR for each client carefully to ensure _____

21. Check _____ date on medication

Down

1. Provide _____ if needed

3. _____ your hands

4. Be sure medications are _____ for each client

6. Prepare meds in a _____ environment

7. Collect all necessary _____

8. Circle _____ and document rationale if drug is not administered

9. Observe client for _____ and document both positive and negative responses

10. Leave client in a position of _____

13. Check need for _____ medications

18. Observe the 5 "_____"

19. Verify all new or questionable orders on the _____ against physician orders for completeness

Principles of Medication Administration

Dr. Evelyn J. Biluk

Word bank

COMFORT   DOSAGE   DRUG   EQUIPMENT   ERRORS   EXPIRATION   IDENTIFIED   INFORM

INITIALS   MAR   PRIVACY   PRN   QUIET   REACTIONS   RIGHTS   SAFETY   THIRTY   THREE

TWO   UNIVERSAL   WASH

Principles of Medication Administration

Dr. Evelyn J. Biluk

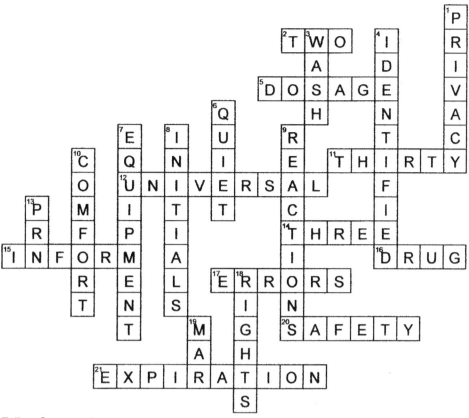

Administration of Oral Medications

Dr. Evelyn J. Biluk

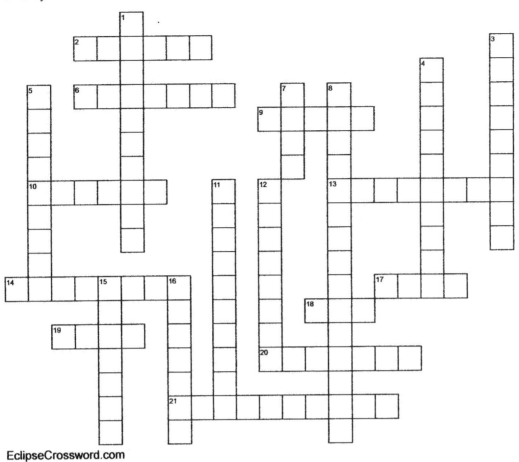

EclipseCrossword.com

Administration of Oral Medications

Dr. Evelyn J. Biluk

Across

2. _____ tablets can be broken

6. Sit client _____ to enhance swallowing

9. Have client use a _____ to prevent staining of teeth by medications that contain iron or HCl

10. Shake _____ meds if necessary to mix

13. _____ containers can remain in their original individual package

14. Read liquid amount at _____ level of med cup at eye level

17. Wipe lip of bottle with _____ towel to prevent stickiness

18. Place all solid meds in _____ medicine cup unless an assessment needs to be made before administration

19. Pour _____ from bottle label

20. _____-coated tablets do not need to be crushed

21. Use _____ dropper, nipple or syringe to give meds to an infant

Down

1. Keep infant at _____ angle during med administration

3. Use agency _____ to crush tablets

4. Use _____ (if possible) for a child or client that is unable to swallow solids

5. Assess client's _____ level, diet status, oral cavity and ability to swallow

7. _____ with client until medication is gone

8. _____ can be mixed with food (exception: Time-release capsules)

11. _____ route has a high rate of absorption

12. Do not use a child's _____ food to administer oral meds

15. Have client _____ medication except with SL route, buccal route, iron or HCL meds

16. If using an NG or _____ tube, check for correct placement before administration and follow medication with water

Administration of Oral Medications

Dr. Evelyn J. Biluk

Word bank

AWAY   CALIBRATED   CAPSULECONTENTS   DAMP   ENTERIC   EQUIPMENT   FAVORITE

FOURTYFIVE   KNOWLEDGE   LIQUID   LIQUIDFORM   MENISCUS   ONE   SCORED   STAY

STOMACH   STRAW   SUBLINGUAL   SWALLOW   UNITDOSE   UPRIGHT

Administration of Oral Medications

Dr. Evelyn J. Biluk

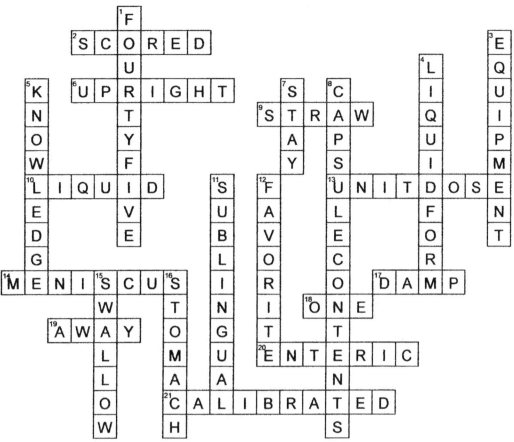

EclipseCrossword.com

Administration of Rectal Drugs

Dr. Evelyn J. Biluk

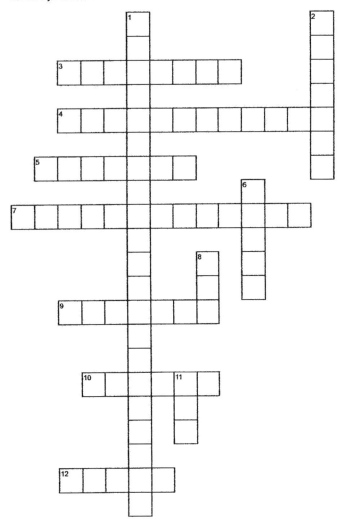

Administration of Rectal Drugs

Dr. Evelyn J. Biluk

Across

3.   Hold client's _____ together after insertion of rectal drug

4.   Remove suppository from _____

5.   Provide _____ to client during procedure

7.   Position client _____

9.   _____ suppository with water-soluble lubricant

10.   If rectal drug is administered as enema, have client retain solution for twenty to _____ minutes

12.   Assess client's _____ function, ability to retain suppository or enema

Down

1.   Suppository needs to pass this anatomical structure

2.   Insert suppository _____ end first

6.   Use _____ or finger cot

8.   Encourage client to retain suppository for _____ to twenty minutes to encourage melting

11.   Insert suppository approximately _____ inches into rectum

Administration of Rectal Drugs

Dr. Evelyn J. Biluk

Word bank

BOWEL   BUTTOCKS   GLOVE   INTERNALANALSPHINCTER   LEFTLATERALLY   MOISTEN   PRIVACY
REFRIGERATOR   TAPERED   TEN   THIRTY   TWO

Administration of Rectal Drugs

Dr. Evelyn J. Biluk

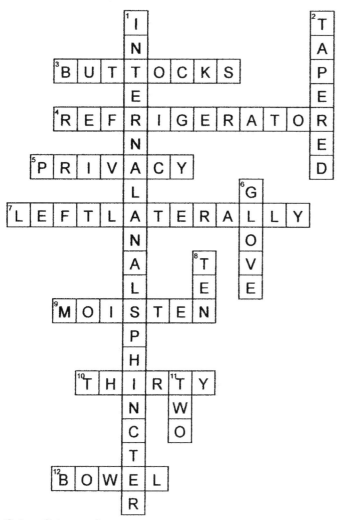

EclipseCrossword.com

Administration of Nasal Medications

Dr. Evelyn J. Biluk

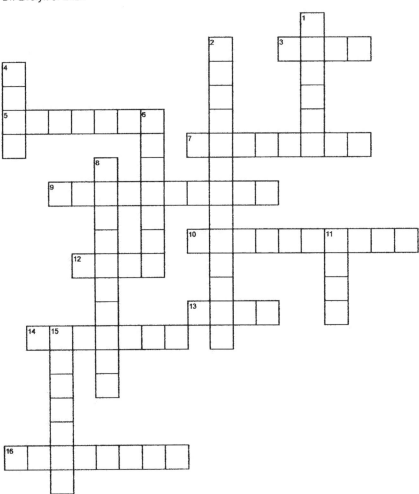

Administration of Nasal Medications

Dr. Evelyn J. Biluk

Across

3. Instruct client to _____ nose

5. Position client in specific position to reach _____

7. If client aspirates and begins to cough, stay with client until _____ is relieved

9. Nasal drops may produce an _____ taste

10. Position client so head can be _____

12. Ask client to keep head tilted for _____ minutes after administration of nasal meds

13. If client is an infant that aspirates and begins to cough, lay infant on his/her _____

14. _____ correct number of drops

16. Place dropper or _____ angled slightly upward just inside nostril

Down

1. Leave kleenex _____ with client

2. Position client's head to aid in _____

4. _____ up on tip of nostril

6. _____ atomizer quickly and firmly

8. Be careful not to touch client's nose with _____

11. Have client _____ nose in order to clear any mucus before med administration

15. Instruct client to _____ to allow for absorption

Administration of Nasal Medications

Dr. Evelyn J. Biluk

Word bank

APPLICATOR   ATOMIZER   BACK   BLOW   DISTRESS   FIVE   GRAVITATIONAL   INSTILL

NOTBLOW   PUSH   SINUSES   SQUEEZE   TILTEDBACK   TISSUE   UNPLEASANT   WIPE

Administration of Nasal Medications

Dr. Evelyn J. Biluk

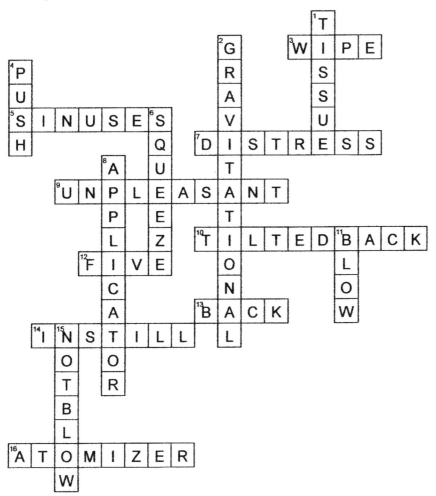

Administration of Inhalants

Dr. Evelyn J. Biluk

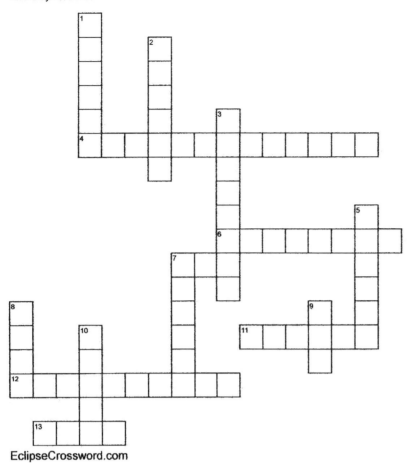

Administration of Inhalants

Dr. Evelyn J. Biluk

Across

4. Encourage _____ of sputum

6. Instruct client to inhale medication until his/her lungs are fully _____

7. After inhalation is complete, have client close his/her mouth and hold their breath for _____ seconds and then exhale

11. Ask client to inhale _____ and deeply while the healthcare provider depressed the canister top

12. Have client place his/her lips around the _____ without touching

13. Client will need to remove the mouthpiece after administration of meds and _____ breath for as long as possible before exhaling completely

Down

1. Have kleenex _____ handy for client

2. A specifically designed _____ device is available to help a client who may have difficulty with the normal inhalant procedure for meds

3. Let client know that _____ is expected after inhalant treatment

5. Have client inhale and exhale _____

7. The _____ can cause inadequate dosing and irritation if inhaler placement is incorrect

8. Wash the client's mouthpiece with _____ water

9. Allow _____ to five minutes between inhalations if procedure needs to be repeated

10. Monitor _____ signs before and after inhalant treatment

Administration of Inhalants

Dr. Evelyn J. Biluk

Word bank

COUGHING   DEEPLY   EXPECTORATION   HOLD   INFLATED   MOUTHPIECE   SLOWLY   SPACER

TEN   TISSUE   TONGUE   TWO   VITAL   WARM

Administration of Inhalants

Dr. Evelyn J. Biluk

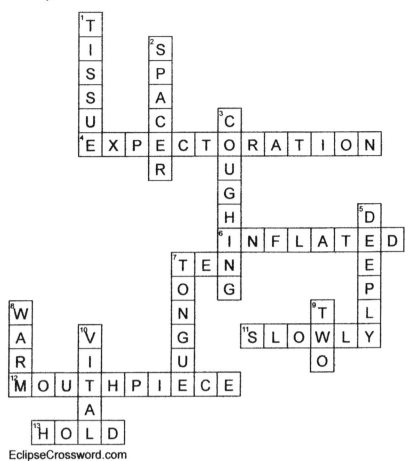

EclipseCrossword.com

Administration of Ophthalmic Medications

Dr. Evelyn J. Biluk

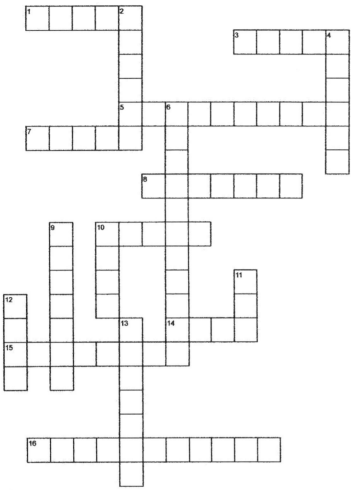

Administration of Ophthalmic Medications

Dr. Evelyn J. Biluk

Across

1. Check solution for _____ before administering
3. Place required number of _____ into lower conjunctiva
5. Do not touch client's eye with _____
7. _____ ointment tube to break medication stream
8. Check solution for _____ before administering
10. Have client _____ two to three times
14. _____ away any excess medication starting from the inner canthus
15. _____ infants and children during administration if necessary
16. Be sure lower _____ is exposed during procedure

Down

2. _____ procedure if necessary using clean tissue
4. Ophthalmic meds should not be _____ between clients
6. Assist client in keeping eye open by _____ on cheekbone
9. _____ eyelid and eyelashes with sterile gauze with physiologic saline
10. Have client lie on _____ or sit with head turned to affected side to aid in gravitational flow
11. Assess _____ condition
12. _____ solution between hands before administration
13. If using ointment, squeeze into lower conjunctiva moving from the inner to the outer _____

Administration of Ophthalmic Medications

Dr. Evelyn J. Biluk

Word bank

APPLICATOR   BACK   BLINK   CANTHUS   CLARITY   CLEANSE   COLOR   CONJUNCTIVA   DROPS
EYE   PULLINGDOWN   REPEAT   RESTRAIN   SHARED   TWIST   WARM   WIPE

Administration of Ophthalmic Medications

Dr. Evelyn J. Biluk

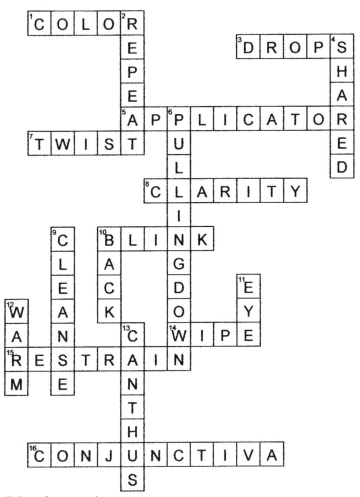

EclipseCrossword.com

Administration of Otic Medications

Dr. Evelyn J. Biluk

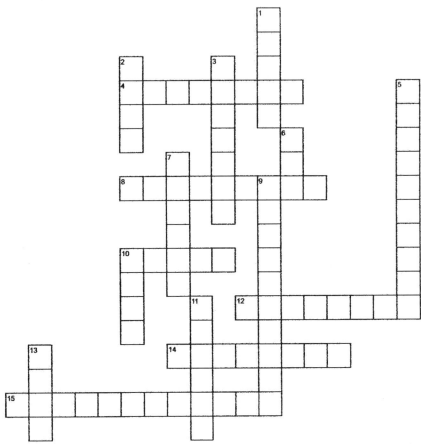

Administration of Otic Medications

Dr. Evelyn J. Biluk

Across

4. Medication needs to reach the _____
8. Repeat _____ if necessary for the other ear
10. Instill correct number of _____ along side of canal
12. _____ infants if necessary; Also children if necessary during procedure
14. Maintain _____ of ear until all medication has entered the ear canal
15. Cotton must be _____ with medication (if being used to keep medication in ear canal)

Down

1. _____ outer ear with a wet gauze
2. Ask client to remain on side for _____ to ten minutes
3. Do not touch ear with dropper
5. _____ ear canal by pulling pinna up and back for adults
6. Assess _____ condition
7. _____ can be used to keep medication in the ear canal
9. Ask client to turn to _____ side to aid in gravitational flow
10. Straighten ear canal by pulling down and _____ for infants and children under 3 yoa
11. Put on _____
13. _____ otic meds in hands before administration

Administration of Otic Medications

Dr. Evelyn J. Biluk

Word bank

CLEAN   COTTON   DOWN   DROPPER   DROPS   EAR   FIVE   GLOVES   INNEREAR   POSITION

PREMOISTENED   PROCEDURE   RESTRAIN   STRAIGHTEN   UNAFFECTED   WARM

Administration of Otic Medications

Dr. Evelyn J. Biluk

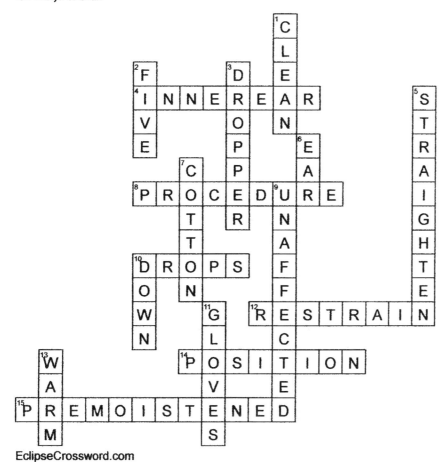

Administration of Topical Agents

Dr. Evelyn J. Biluk

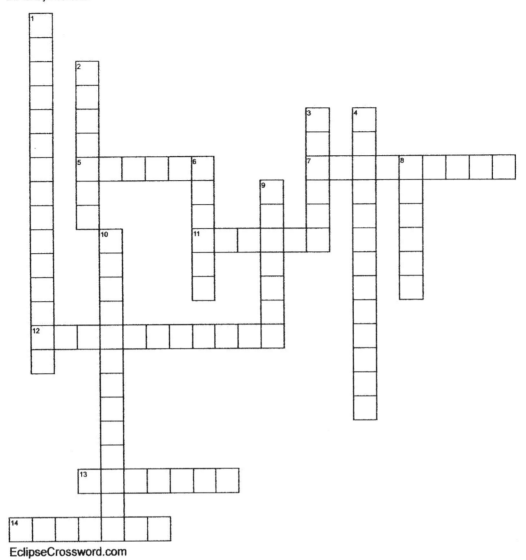

Administration of Topical Agents

Dr. Evelyn J. Biluk

Across

5. Use _____ and gauze, tongue depressor or sterile applicator, if integument is broken

7. When using _____ patches, use gloves

11. _____ only appropriate area of client to promote comfort

12. Applying medication offers an _____ to talke about client's problems and share information about improvements

13. Provide the client with _____

14. _____ area of old medications using gauze pads with soap and warm water

Down

1. Use gloves to prevent _____ during administration

2. Assess area for any _____

3. Remove backing and place transderm patch in area with _____ hair

4. Clients often receive topical agents for _____ problems

6. _____ medication over site evenly and thinly

8. Press edges of transderm patch down to _____ patch

9. If necessary, cover area _____ with a dressing

10. When applying _____ ointment, take clients BP for five minutes before and after application

Administration of Topical Agents

Dr. Evelyn J. Biluk

Word bank

CHANGES   CLEANSE   EXPOSE   GLOVES   IMAGEALTERING   LITTLE   LOOSELY   NITROGLYCERIN

OPPORTUNITY   PRIVACY   SECURE   SELF-ABSORPTION   SPREAD   TRANSDERM

Administration of Topical Agents

Dr. Evelyn J. Biluk

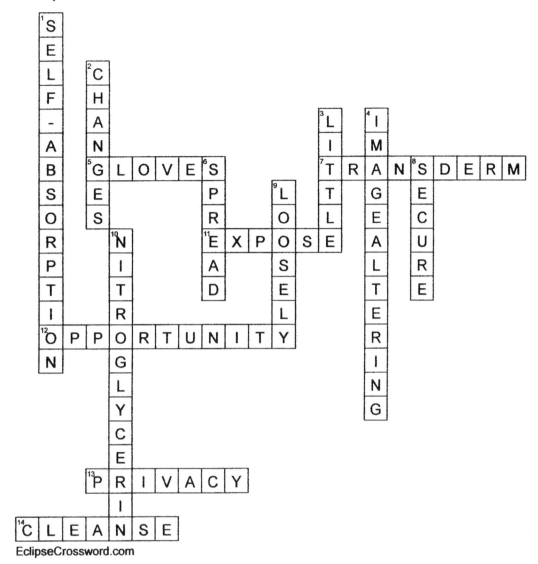

EclipseCrossword.com

Administration of Vaginal Medications

Dr. Evelyn J. Biluk

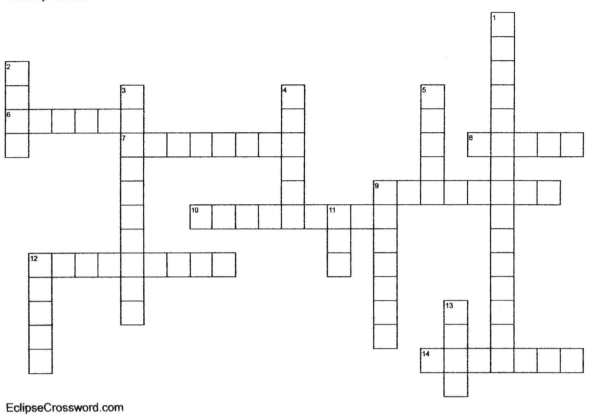

EclipseCrossword.com

Administration of Vaginal Medications

Dr. Evelyn J. Biluk

Across

6. If giving _____, dry client's buttocks

7. Angle applicator _____ and back

8. Use _____ during administration of vaginal medications

9. Cleanse _____ with warm, soapy water

10. There is no _____ to hold the suppository in place for client

12. Moisten applicator tip with water-soluble _____ or just water

14. Have client remain in position for about _____ to twenty minutes

Down

1. Place client in _____ position with hips and knees flexed

2. Provide client with _____ after administration if needed

3. Instill _____

4. Place client on _____

5. Wash applicator when finished with warm, soapy _____

9. Provide client with _____

11. Insert applicator about _____ inches

12. Separate _____ in female client to insert applicator

13. Have client ___ before administration begins

Administration of Vaginal Medications

Dr. Evelyn J. Biluk

Word bank

BEDPAN   DORSALRECUMBENT   DOUCHE   DOWNWARD   FIFTEEN   GLOVE   LABIA   LUBRICANT
MEDICATION   PADS   PERINEUM   PRIVACY   SPHINCTER   TWO   VOID   WATER

Administration of Vaginal Medications

Dr. Evelyn J. Biluk

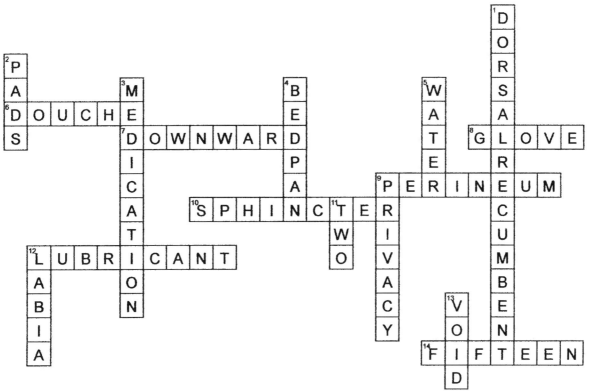

EclipseCrossword.com

Administration of Parenteral Medications

Dr. Evelyn J. Biluk

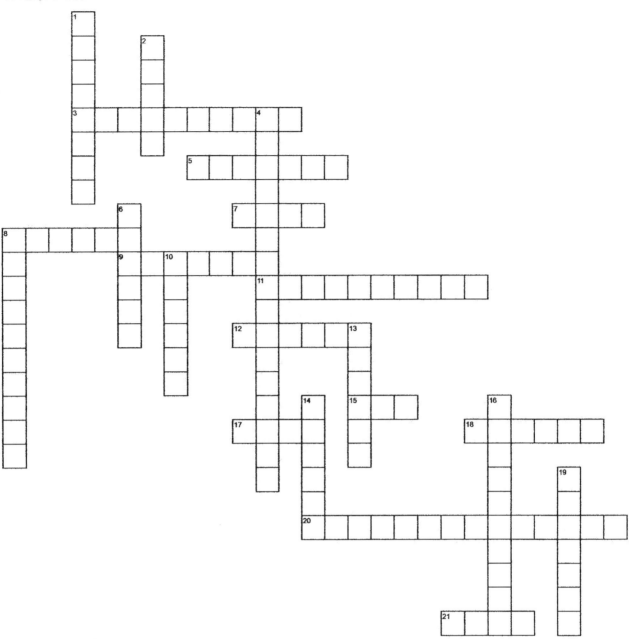

Administration of Parenteral Medications

Dr. Evelyn J. Biluk

Across

3. Use _____ 1 mL syringe for volumes less than 1 mL

5. _____ of syringe in appropriate manner

7. Select appropriate _____

8. When using an _____, tap neck to force medication into ampule

9. Remove needle and _____ area (exception: heparin or a Z-track injection)

11. Assess for _____

12. When mixing a _____, use a filter needle when drawing up medication

15. Without contaminating the plunger, draw up _____ equal to the amount of medication needed

17. When medication comes in a _____, cleanse rubber stopper with alcohol

18. _____ site when documenting medication administration

20. Assess client's ability for _____ if appropriate

21. Assess _____ for presence of lesions, rashes or abscesses prio to administration of parenteral medications

Down

1. Inject the air into the vial to prevent _____ pressure and aid in aspirating medication

2. Replace protective _____ on needle before proceeding

4. Assess client for _____ which may affect side selection

6. _____ the appropriate amount of medication from the vial

8. Check to ensure there are no _____ present

10. Inject medication _____

13. _____ sites as much as possible

14. Wear _____ to avoid contact with blood

16. Select appropriate _____ and syringe

19. Insert needle _____ with bevel up

Administration of Parenteral Medications

Dr. Evelyn J. Biluk

Word bank

AIR   AIRBUBBLES   AMPULE   AREA   COVER   DISCOMFORT   DISPOSE   GLOVES

IMPAIREDMOBILITY   MASSAGE   NEEDLESIZE   NEGATIVE   POWDER   QUICKLY   RECORD

REMOVE   ROTATE   SELF-INJECTION   SITE   SLOWLY   TUBERCULIN   VIAL

Administration of Parenteral Medications

Dr. Evelyn J. Biluk

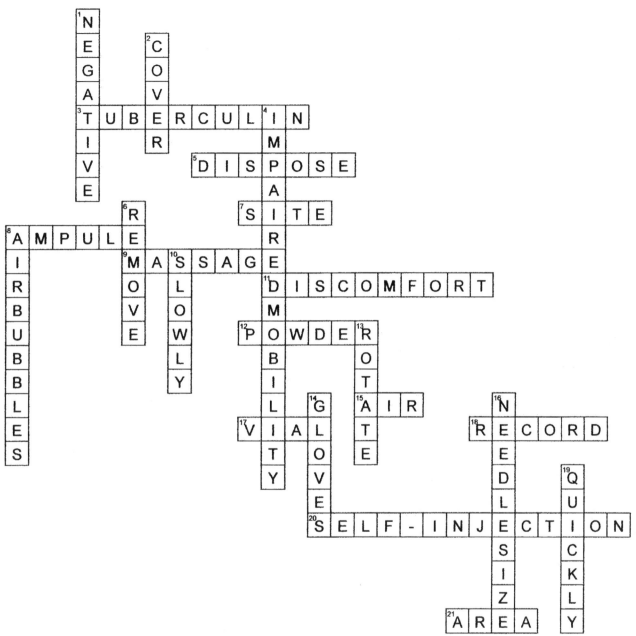

Local Anesthetics

Dr. Evelyn J. Biluk

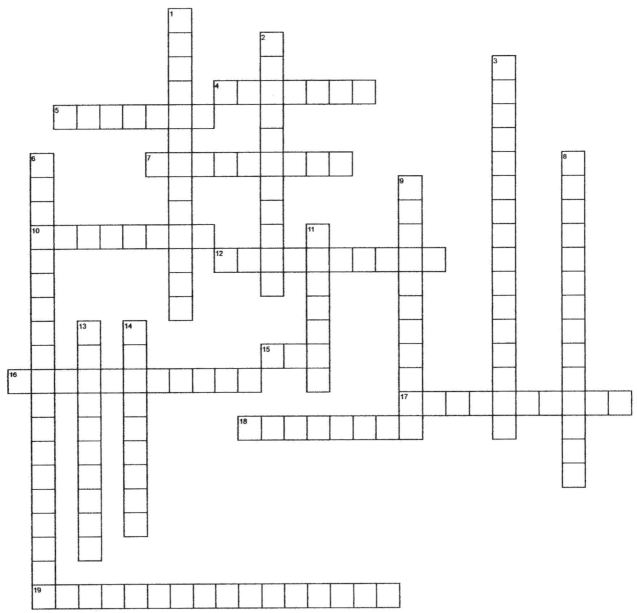

Local Anesthetics

Dr. Evelyn J. Biluk

Across

4. Benzocaine is used for _____ anesthesia

5. _____ effects of local anesthetics include drowsiness, dizziness, lightheadedness, restlessness, numbness of lips and tongue, headache with spinal anesthesia, hypotension, bradycardia, cardiovascular collapse, convulsions, tinnitus, muscle weakness, anaphylaxis and respiratory depression

7. AKA Xylocaine

10. _____ is seen more often with bupivacaine in children and elderly

12. AKA Americaine

15. Benzocaine is commonly found in _____ preparations to treat sunburns, rashes, sore throats and hemorrhoids

16. AKA Marcaine

17. Mepivacaine is used for infiltration _____ anesthesia

18. AKA Novocain

19. Procaine is used for nerve block, _____ and infiltration anesthesia

Down

1. Emergency _____ equipment should be made available for clients on procaine

2. AKA Carbocaine

3. Viscous lidocaine can interfere with _____ and clients should wait at least 60 minutes after use before eating

6. Etidocaine is used for infiltration anesthesia, peripheral nerve block and _____

8. Bupivacaine is used for _____, infiltration anesthesia and peripheral nerve block

9. _____ prolongs anesthetic action, while shortening the onset of action and reducing blood flow to injection site

11. Mepivacaine has 2 times the _____ and toxicity of lidocaine

13. AKA Duranest

14. _____ effects last 1.5 to 2 times longer with etidocaine than lidocaine

Local Anesthetics

Dr. Evelyn J. Biluk

Word bank

ADVERSE   ANALGESIA   BENZOCAINE   BUPIVACAINE   CENTRALNEURALBLOCKS   EPIDURALBLOCKS

EPINEPHRINE   ETIDOCAINE   LIDOCAINE   MEPIVACAINE   NERVEBLOCK   OTC   POTENCY

PROCAINE   RESUSCITATION   SPINALANESTHESIA   SWALLOWINGREFLEX   TOPICAL   TOXICITY

Local Anesthetics

Dr. Evelyn J. Biluk

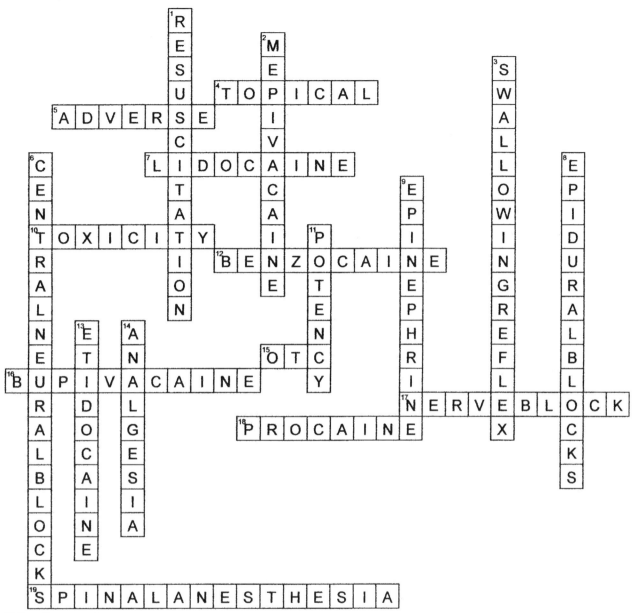

Nonnarcotic Analgesics and Antipyretics

Dr. Evelyn J. Biluk

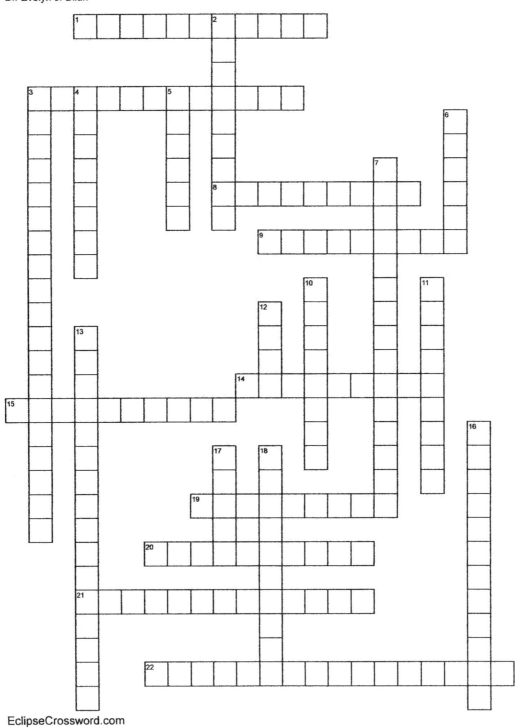

Nonnarcotic Analgesics and Antipyretics

Dr. Evelyn J. Biluk

Across

1. Inhibits formation of prostaglandins in production of fever; Acts on the hypothalamus to produce vasodilation

3. Occurs when aspirin inhibits prostaglandin derivative, thromboxane A2

8. AKA Motrin, Advil

9. AKA Feldene

14. AKA Toradol

15. Indocine may cause _____, anorexia, severe headache, corneal cloudiness and visual field changes

19. Inhibits the formation of prostaglandins involved with pain; Occurs by action of hypothalamus and blocking generation of pain impulses

20. Feldene can cause a higher incidence of _____

21. AKA Tylenol

22. Adverse effects of tylenol include rash, _____ and liver toxicity

Down

2. AKA Vioxx

3. AKA Aspirin

4. Adverse effects of salicylates include tinnitus, confusion and dizziness

5. Bextra may cause _____, fluid retention or increased BP

6. Ibuprofen may cause _____ or water retention

7. Celebrex may cause _____, abdominal pain or an upper respiratory infection

10. AKA Naprosyn

11. AKA Celebrex

12. Toradol cannot be given to a client for longer than _____ days

13. Inhibits prostaglandin synthesis causing _____ action

16. AKA Indocin

17. Toradol has an increased risk of _____ impairment and GI bleeding in prolonged use

18. AKA Bextra

Nonnarcotic Analgesics and Antipyretics

Dr. Evelyn J. Biluk

Word bank

ACETAMINOPHEN   ACETYLSALICYLICACID   ANALGESIA   ANEMIA   ANTIINFLAMMATORY

ANTIPLATELET   ANTIPYRETIC   CELECOXIB   FIVE   GIBLEEDING   GIDISTRESS   IBUPROFEN

INDOMETHACIN   KETOROLAC   NAPROXEN   PERIPHERALEDEMA   PIROXICAM   RENAL   ROFECOXIB

SODIUM   THROMBOCYTOPENIA   TINNITUS   VALDECOXIB

Nonnarcotic Analgesics and Antipyretics

Dr. Evelyn J. Biluk

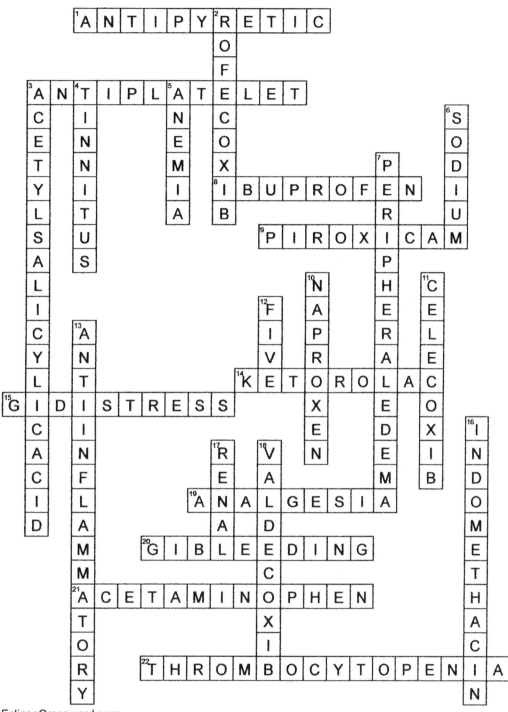

Narcotic Analgesics

Dr. Evelyn J. Biluk

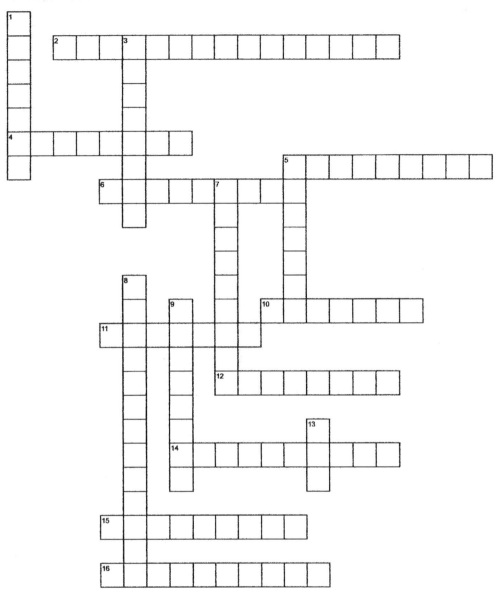

Narcotic Analgesics

Dr. Evelyn J. Biluk

Across

2. Acts on opioid receptors in CNS; Induces sedation, analgesia and euphoria; Provide pain relief in MI; Relief of moderate to severe pain

4. AKA Narcan; Narcotic antagonist

5. AKA Methadone

6. Used for severe pain; Narcotic withdrawal; IM preferred route

10. _____ should not be taken with narcotic analgesics

11. _____ effects of narcotic analgesics include sedation, confusion, euphoria, impaired coordination, dizziness, urinary retention, constipation, hyperglycemia, respiratory depression, hypotension, tachycardia, bradycardia, nausea, vomiting, decreased uterine contractility, allergic reactions, tolerance, physical and psychological dependence and pupil constriction

12. AKA Hydromorphone

14. Narcotic _____ can reverse the effects of a narcotic analgesic if necessary

15. A larger dose of narcotic analgesic is required to produce the original effect

16. Used for moderate to sever pain; Preoperative medication; PO dose < 50 % as effective as parenteral; IM preferred route for duplicate doses

Down

1. Used for moderate to sever pain; Cough relief; Smoking can reduce pain relief

3. AKA Percodan, Oxycodone Hydrochloride

5. AKA Meperidine

7. First sign of tolerance is usually a _____ duration of effect of the analgesic

8. Used for moderate to severe pain; Mix with 5 mL of sterile water or normal saline for IV use; Smoking reduces pain relief

9. Used for moderate to severe pain; Monitor liver and blood studies; Give oral form with food; High abuse potential

13. _____ depressants should not be taken with narcotic analgesics

Narcotic Analgesics

Dr. Evelyn J. Biluk

Word bank

ADVERSE   ALCOHOL   ANTAGONIST   CNS   CODEINE   DECREASED   DEMEROL   DILAUDID

DOLOPHINE   HYDROMORPHONE   MEPERIDINE   METHADONE   MORPHINESULFATE   NALOXONE

PERCOCET   PERCODAN   TOLERANCE

Narcotic Analgesics

Dr. Evelyn J. Biluk

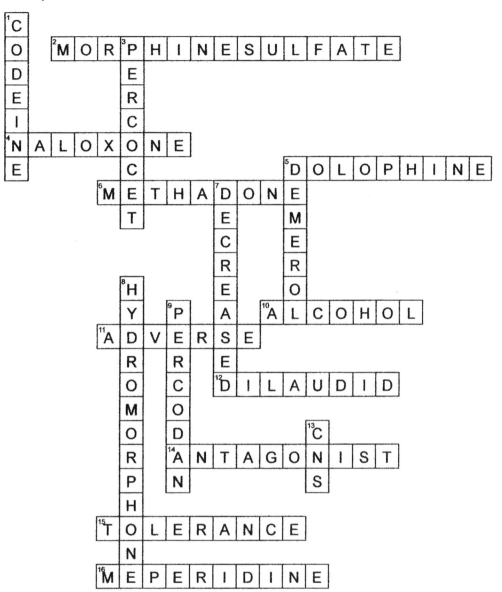

Narcotic Antagonists

Dr. Evelyn J. Biluk

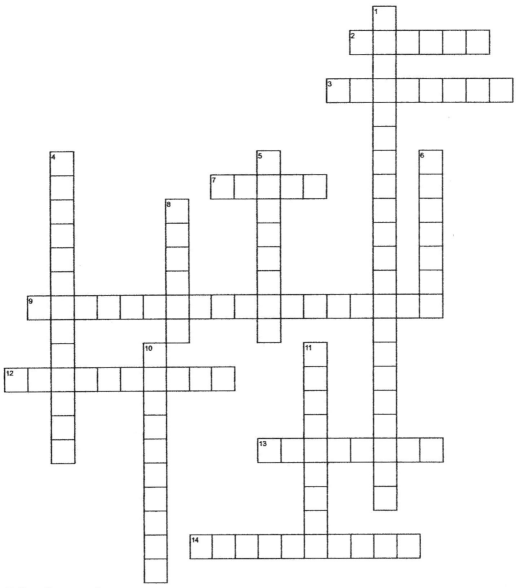

Narcotic Antagonists

Dr. Evelyn J. Biluk

Across

2. AKA Naloxone Hydrochloride

3. Narcan occupies opiate receptor sites and prevents or reverses effects of _____ such as morphine sulfate

7. AKA Nalmefene

9. _____ can be experienced in clients addicted to narcotics that are given naloxone hydrochloride

12. _____ need to be monitored (especially respirations) for clients on naloxone hydrochloride

13. Surgical clients on narcan need to be monitored for _____

14. _____ is used in narcotic detoxification and to prevent readdiction in drug users

Down

1. _____ is used for postoperative respiratory depression caused by narcotics, therapy in suspected or confirmed narcotic overdose

4. Emergency _____ equipment needs to be available for clients on narcan

5. Tremors are an adverse effect of narcan and indicate an _____ of the drug

6. _____ effects of narcan when excess dosage occurs include hypertension, tremors, reversal of analgesia, hyperventilation and increased PTT

8. AKA Naltrexone

10. _____ symptoms will be observed in clients addicted to narcotics

11. _____ is used to treat opioid overdose

Narcotic Antagonists

Dr. Evelyn J. Biluk

Word bank

ADVERSE   AGONISTS   BLEEDING   NALMEFENE   NALOXONEHYDROCHLORIDE   NALTREXONE

NARCAN   OVERDOSE   RESUSCITATIVE   REVEX   TREXAN   VITALSIGNS   WITHDRAWAL

WITHDRAWALSYNDROME

Narcotic Antagonists

Dr. Evelyn J. Biluk

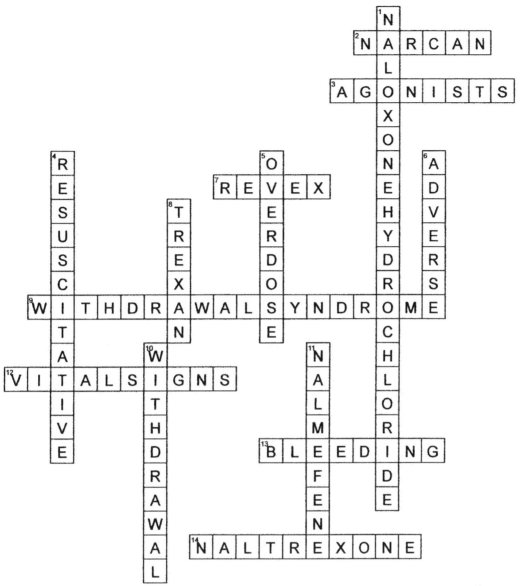

Sedatives and Hypnotics

Dr. Evelyn J. Biluk

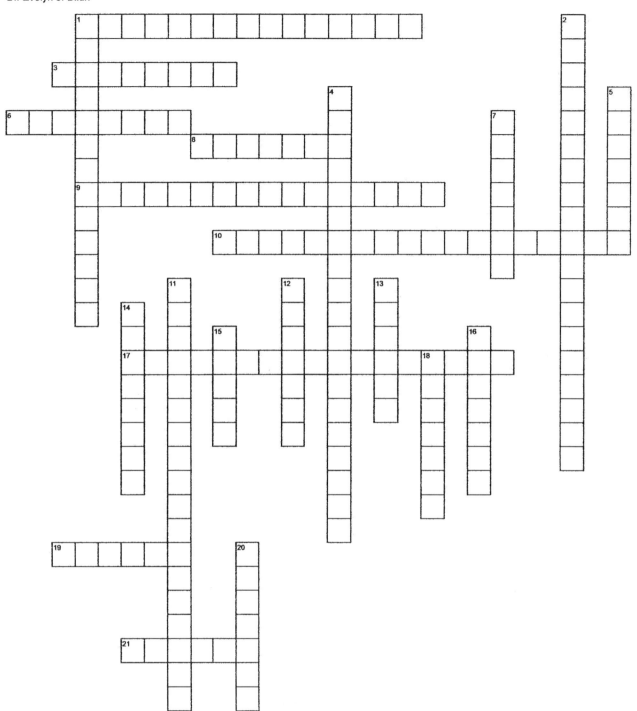

Sedatives and Hypnotics

Dr. Evelyn J. Biluk

Across

1.   AKA Thiopental Sodium

3.   AKA Pentobarbital Sodium

6.   AKA Clonazepam; Used for seizures, restless leg syndrome and panic attacks

8.   AKA Triazolam; Used for hypnosis

9.   Used for induction of general anesthesia, acute seizures, decrease of IC pressure during neurosurgery, narcoanalysis and narcosynthesis in psychiatry; Ultrashort acting barbiturate

10.   Used for sedation, hypnosis, preoperative medication; Intermediate acing barbiturate

17.   Used for sedation, hypnosis, preoperative medication, labor, chronic/acute seizures

19.   AKA Amobarbital Sodium

21.   AKA Lorazepam; Used for anxiety and preoperative medication

Down

1.   _____ should not receive barbiturates

2.   Used for sedation, hypnosis and seizure disorders

4.   Used for sedation, hypnosis, preoperative medication; Short acting barbiturate

5.   AKA Chlordiazepoxide; Used for anxiety and alcohol withdrawal

7.   _____ effects of luminal include dizziness, ataxia, drowsiness, hangover feeling, anxiety, irritability, hand tremors, vision difficulties, insomnia, bradycardia, low BP, chest tightness, wheezing, apnea, respiratory depression, nausea, vomiting, constipation, hypersensitivity reactions

11.   Used for hypnosis, preoperative medication; Short acting barbiturate

12.   AKA Butabarbital Sodium

13.   AKA Midazolam; Used for preoperative medication and conscious sedation

14.   AKA Chlorazepate; Used for anxiety

15.   AKA Alprazolam; Used for anxiety

16.   AKA Phenobarbital Sodium

18.   AKA Flurazepam; Used for hypnosis

20.   AKA Secobarbital Sodium

Sedatives and Hypnotics

Dr. Evelyn J. Biluk

Word bank

ADVERSE   AMOBARBITALSODIUM   AMYTAL   ATIVAN   BUTABARBITALSODIUM   BUTISOL   DALMANE

HALCION   KLONOPIN   LIBRIUM   LUMINAL   NEMBUTAL   PENTOBARBITALSODIUM

PENTOTHALSODIUM   PHENOBARBITALSODIUM   PREGNANTWOMEN   SECOBARBITALSODIUM

SECONAL   THIOPENTALSODIUM   TRANXENE   VERSED   XANAX

Sedatives and Hypnotics

Dr. Evelyn J. Biluk

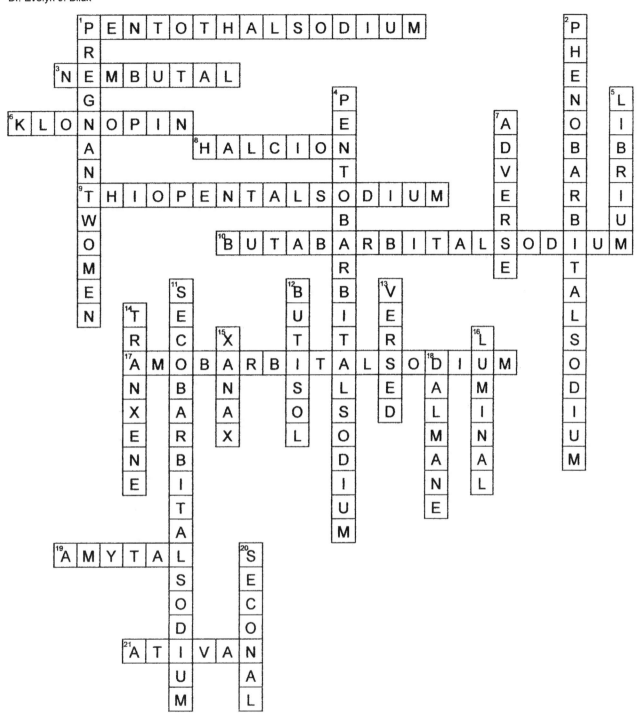

EclipseCrossword.com

Anticonvulsants

Dr. Evelyn J. Biluk

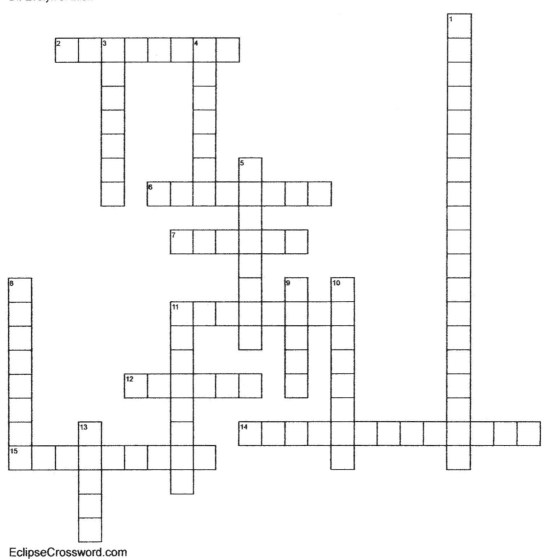

Anticonvulsants

Dr. Evelyn J. Biluk

Across

2. _____ is the drug of choice for status epilepticus

6. AKA Felbamate; Used to treat Lennox-Gastaut Syndrome in children and partial seizures

7. AKA Diazepam; Used for status epilepticus and absence seizures; Category: Benzodiazepines

11. AKA Valproic Acid; Used in treatment of absence seizures; Category: Adjunct anticonvulsants

12. AKA Acetazolamide; Diuretic used as an adjunct or alone in treatment of absence, tonic-clonic or myoclonic seizures

14. Used for generalized and absence seizures; Category: Barbiturates

15. AKA Gabapentin; Used to treat partial seizures

Down

1. _____ is seen most often in children and adolescents

3. _____ effects of hydantoins include confusion, slurred speech, slow physical movment, blood dyscrasias, nausea, vomiting, constipation, gingival hyperplasia, hirsutism, rash, acne, hypotension, circulatory collapse, cardiac arrest

4. _____ use can cause drug toxicity

5. AKA Lamotrigine; Used to treat partial seizures

8. AKA Ethosuximide; Used in treatment of absence seizures; Category: Succinimides

9. May take _____ to ten days to achieve therapeutic serum concentration

10. AKA Carbamazepine; Used in treatment of tonic-clonic, complex partial and mixed seizures

11. AKA Phenytoin; Used for tonic-clonic and complex partial seizures, status epilepticus, prevention of seizures that accompany neurosurgery; Category: Hydantoins

13. _____ may turn pink, red or red-brown while taking hydantoins

Anticonvulsants

Dr. Evelyn J. Biluk

Word bank

ADVERSE   ALCOHOL   DEPAKENE   DIAMOX   DIAZEPAM   DILANTIN   FELBATOL

GINGIVALHYPERPLASIA   LAMICTAL   NEURONTIN   PHENOBARBITAL   SEVEN   TEGRETOL   URINE

VALIUM   ZARONTIN

Anticonvulsants

Dr. Evelyn J. Biluk

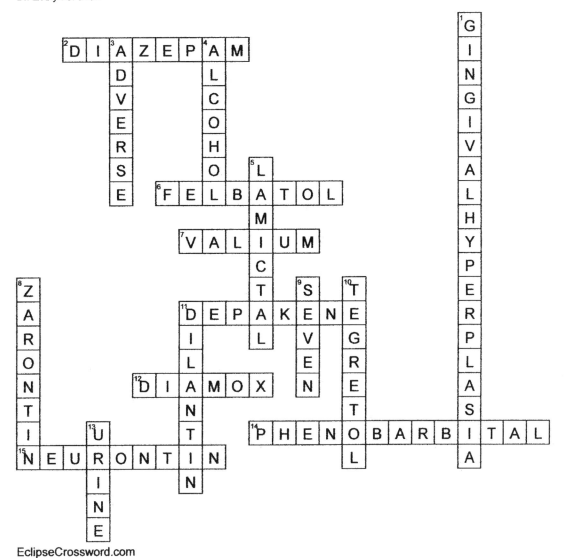

Muscle Relaxants

Dr. Evelyn J. Biluk

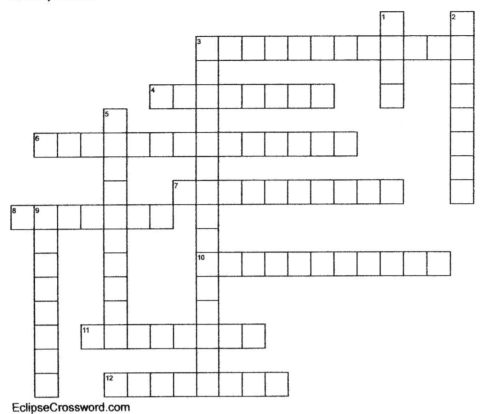

Muscle Relaxants

Dr. Evelyn J. Biluk

Across

3. Used in cerebral palsy, muscle stiffness and aspsm found in a variety of musculoskeletal disorders

4. Used in multiple sclerosis and spinal cord injuries

6. Adverse effects of dantrium include drowsiness, malaise, diarrhea, and _____

7. The _____ effects of lioresal may increase if mixed with other CNS depressants

8. _____ effects of lioresal include CNS depression (ranging from sedation to comma and seizures), urinary frequency, hirsutism, photosensitivity, acne-like rash, nausea and vomiting

10. Adverse effects of flexeril include _____, dizziness, drowsiness, confusion, fatigue, headache, nervousness, blurred vision, constipation, dyspepsia, nausea, unpleasant taste and urinary retention

11. Adverse effects of soma include _____, headache, syncope, tachycardia, postural hypotension, nausea, vomiting, hiccups and allergic reactions

12. AKA Baclofen

Down

1. AKA Carisoprodol

2. AKA Cyclobenzaprine

3. Used for managing acute and painful muscle spasm

5. Used for muscle spasms associated with CVA, spinal cord injury, cerebral palsy and multiple sclerosis; Given intravenously for malignant hyperthermia

9. AKA Dantrolene

Muscle Relaxants

Dr. Evelyn J. Biluk

Word bank

ADVERSE   ARRHYTHMIAS   BACLOFEN   CARISOPRODOL   CYCLOBENZAPRINE   DANTRIUM

DANTROLENE   DEPRESSANT   FLEXERIL   HEPATOTOXICITY   LIORESAL   SEDATION   SOMA

Muscle Relaxants

Dr. Evelyn J. Biluk

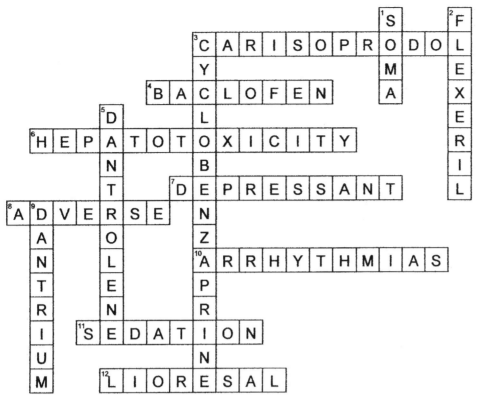

EclipseCrossword.com

Antipsychotic Agents I

Dr. Evelyn J. Biluk

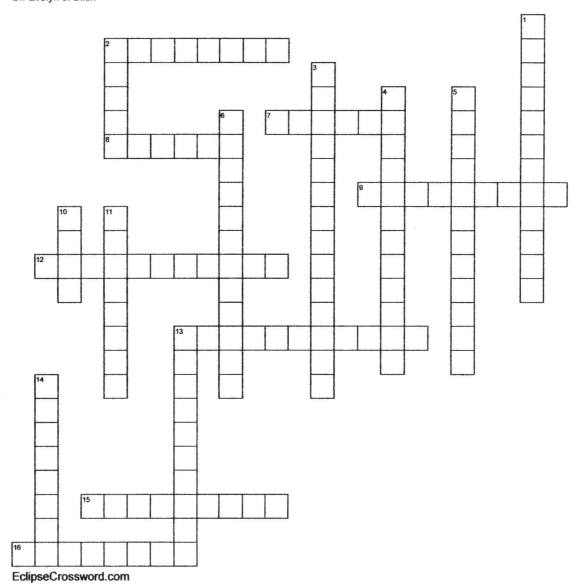

Antipsychotic Agents I

Dr. Evelyn J. Biluk

Across

2. AKA Thioridazine

7. AKA Haloperidol

8. AKA Thiothixene

9. AKA Promethazine

12. Used for psychotic disorders, Tourette's syndrome and short term treatment in hyperactive children

13. Used for psychotic disorders; Clients at great risk for extrapyramidal symptoms; AKA Navane

15. Used for psychotic disorders; Clients at low risk for sedation and extrapyramidal symptoms; AKA Moban

16. AKA Mesoridazine

Down

1. Used for psychotic disorders, attention deficit disorder and short term use in depression

2. AKA Molindone

3. Used for management of acute and chronic schizophrenia, manic phase of bipolar disorder, management of nause and vomiting, control of excessive anxiety before surgery, treatment of acute intermittent porphyria, treatment of intractable hiccups and tetanus

4. Used for psychotic disorders; Clients at great risk for extrapyramidal symptoms

5. Used for preoperative and postoperative sedation, prophylaxis for nausea, vomiting, motion sickness and adjunct to analgesics and allergic conditions

6. Used for schizophrenia and acute/chronic alcoholism; AKA Serentil

10. AKA Pimozide

11. AKA Fluphenazine

13. AKA Chlorpromazine; Category: Phenothiazines

14. Used for Tourette's Syndrome; Decreased sedation

Antipsychotic Agents I

Dr. Evelyn J. Biluk

Word bank

CHLORPROMAZINE   FLUPHENAZINE   HALDOL   HALOPERIDOL   MELLARIL   MESORIDAZINE

MOBAN   MOLINDONE   NAVANE   ORAP   PHENERGAN   PIMOZIDE   PROLIXIN   PROMETHAZINE

SERENTIL   THIORIDAZINE   THIOTHIXENE   THORAZINEL

Antipsychotic Agents I

Dr. Evelyn J. Biluk

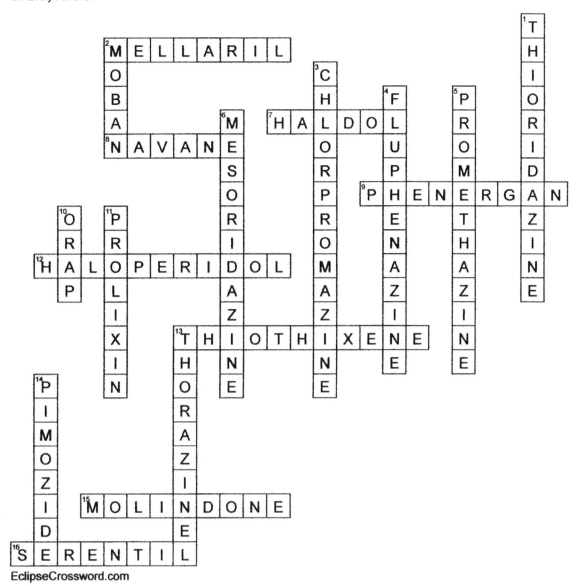

EclipseCrossword.com

Antipsychotic Agents II

Dr. Evelyn J. Biluk

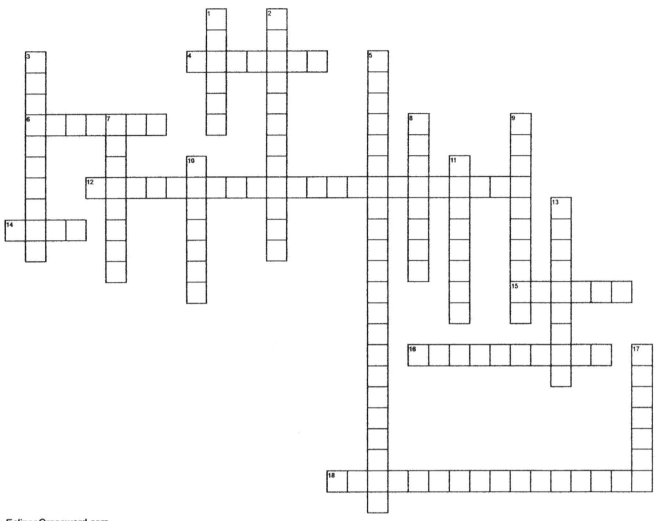

Antipsychotic Agents II

Dr. Evelyn J. Biluk

Across

4. AKA Isocarboxazid; Category: MAO Inhibitor

6. AKA Nortriptyline

12. Adverse effects of MAO inhibitors include _____, dry mouth, blurred vision, constipation, hypertensive crisis, liver dysfunction and leukopenia

14. Clients need to maintain sodium intake of _____ g per day to prevent lithium toxicity

15. AKA Phenelzine; Category: MAO Inhibitor

16. Used for endogenous and reactive depression as well as childhood enuresis

18. Used for treatment and prophylaxis of manic phase of bipolar disorder

Down

1. AKA Amitriptyline

2. Adverse effects of lithium carbonate include _____, confusion, restlessness, fatigue, weakness, hand tremors, arrhythmias, circulatory collapse, hypotension, blurred vision, dry mouth, thirst, weight gain, nausea, diarrhea and leukocytosis

3. AKA Lithium Citrate

5. Adverse effects of tricyclic antidepressants include _____, sedation, confusion, orthostatic hypotension, arrhythmias, blood dyscrasias, extrapyramidal symptoms, gynecomastia and jaundice

7. AKA Imipramine; Category: Tricyclic Antidepressants

8. AKA Doxepin

9. Used for neurotic and atypical depression

10. AKA Amoxapine

11. AKA Lithium Carbonate

13. AKA Desipramine

17. AKA Tranylcypromine; Contraindicated in clients over 60 yoa; Category: MAO Inhibitor

Antipsychotic Agents II

Dr. Evelyn J. Biluk

Word bank

6-10   ANTICHOLINERGICEFFECTS   ASENDIN   AVENTYL   CIBALITH-S   ELAVIL   ESKALITH

IMIPRAMINE   LITHIUMCARBONATE   MARPLAN   NARDIL   NORPRAMIN   ORTHOSTATICHYPOTENSION

PALPITATIONS   PARNATE   PHENELZINE   SINEQUAN   TOFRANIL

Antipsychotic Agents II

Dr. Evelyn J. Biluk

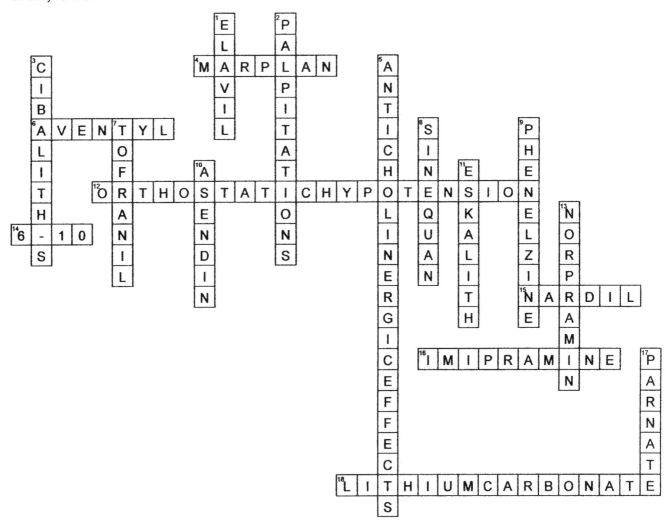

Antipsychotic Agents III

Dr. Evelyn J. Biluk

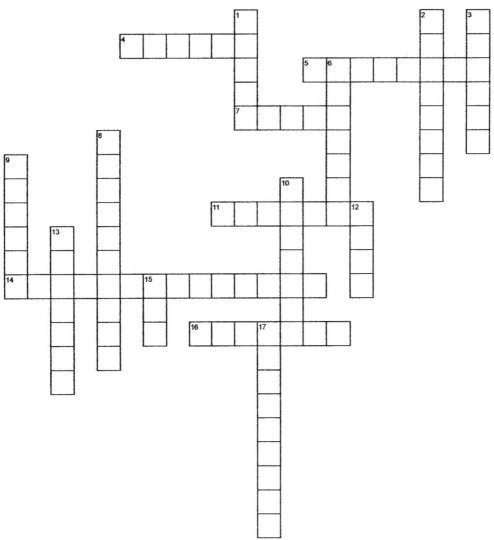

Antipsychotic Agents III

Dr. Evelyn J. Biluk

Across

4. AKA Citalopram

5. AKA Clozapine; Antidepressant

7. AKA Fluvoxamine

11. AKA Venlafaxine; Antidepressant

14. Adverse effects of selective serotonin reuptake inhibitors includes _____, sexual dysfunction, nausea, headache, anorexia, weight loss and skin rash

16. AKA Olanzapine; Antidepressant

Down

1. AKA Paroxetine

2. Prozac interacts with _____

3. AKA Sertraline

6. AKA Escitalopram

8. AKA Buproprion; Antidepressant

9. AKA Fluoxetine; Category: Selective Serotonin Reuptake Inhibitors

10. AKA Nefazodone; Antidepressant

12. A skin _____ resulting from the use of prozac indicates an allergic reaction; Needs to be reported to the physician immediately

13. AKA Trazodone; Antidepressant

15. Prozac cannot be combined with _____ inhibitors

17. AKA Risperidone; Antidepressant

Antipsychotic Agents III

Dr. Evelyn J. Biluk

Word bank

CELEXA   CLOZARIL   CNSSTIMULATION   DESYREL   EFFEXOR   LEXAPRO   LUVOX   MAO   PAXIL

PROZAC   RASH   RISPERDAL   SERZONE   WARFARIN   WELLBUTRIN   ZOLOFT   ZYPREXA

Antipsychotic Agents III
Dr. Evelyn J. Biluk

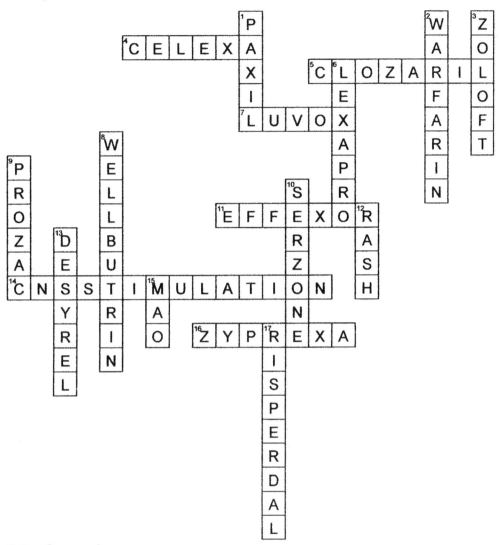

EclipseCrossword.com

Direct Acting Adrenergics

Dr. Evelyn J. Biluk

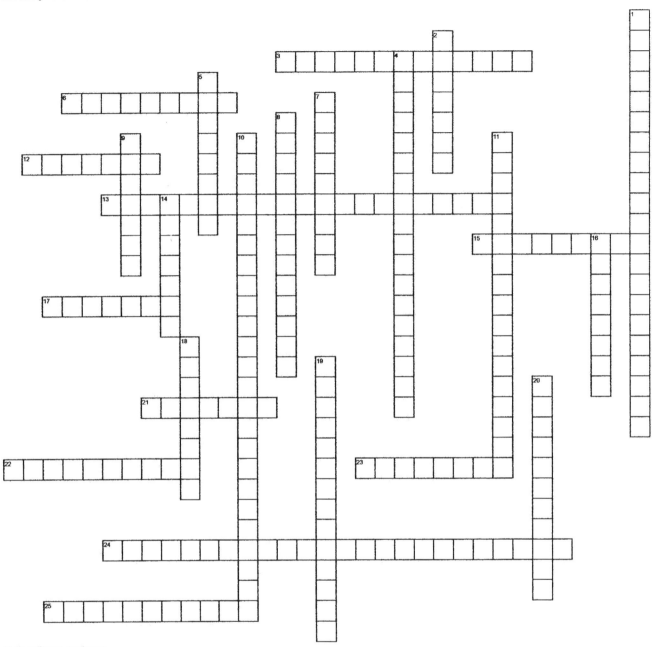

Direct Acting Adrenergics

Dr. Evelyn J. Biluk

Across

3. Used for acute heart failure, management of intraoperative bronchospasm, additive treatment in cardiac arrest, AV heart block, Stokes-Adams syndrome, treatment of chronic bronchoconstriction, management of syncope, treatment of bronchospasm in COPD and asthma

6. Used to relief allergies and mild asthma; Therapy in shock and hypotension; Actions similar to the peripheral autonomic effects of norepinephrine

12. AKA Ritodrine; Nonselective Beta Agonist

13. Used to correct hemodynamic imbalance in shock caused by MI, trauma, septicemia, CHF and open heart surgery

15. AKA Isoxsuprine Hydrochloride; Nonselective Beta Agonists

17. AKA Metaproterenol Sulfate; Selective Beta-2 Agonist

21. AKA Isoproterenol; Nonselective Beta (Beta-1 and Beta-2) Agonists

22. Used in treatment of acute heart failure; Given to adults via IV infusion; Selective Beta-1 Agonist

23. AKA Terbutaline Sulfate; Selective Beta-2 Agonist

24. Used in cerebrovascular insufficiency and peripheral vascular disease; Nonselective Beta Agonist

25. Used for treating acute hypotension seen during surgery

Down

1. Used to treat bronchial asthma and bronchospasm that accompanies emphysema and bronchitis

2. AKA Metaraminol; Used for acute hypotension and can be given preoperatively to prevent hypotension

4. AKA Brethine

5. AKA Dopamine Hydrochloride; Selective Beta-1 Agonist

7. Used for management of preterm labor; Nonselective Beta Agonist

8. Used to stabilize BP during anesthesia, vascular failure in shock, subdues paroxysmal supraventricular tachycardia, rhinitis of allergy and common cold, sinusitis, wide-angle glaucoma and ophthalmoscopic exam or surgery and uveitis; Selective Alpha Agonist

9. AKA Methoxamine; Selective Alpha Agonists

10. Used to revive BP in acute hypotensive states; Adjunct in treatment of cardiac arrest; Nonselective (Alpha and Beta) Agonists

11. AKA Epinephrine; Nonselective (Alpha and Beta) Agonists

14. Adverse effects of epinephrine include _____, headache, fear, arrhythmias, hypertension, cerebral/subarachnoid hemorrhage, hemiplegia, pulmonary edema, insomnia, anginal pain in clients with angina pectoris, tremors, vertigo, sweating, nausea, vomiting, agitation, disorientation, paranoid delusions

16. AKA Norepinephrine Bitartrate; Nonselective (Alpha and Beta) Agonists

18. AKA Dobutamine; Selective Beta-1 Agonist

19. AKA Phenylephrine; Selective Alpha Agonists

20. Adverse effects of levophed include _____, cardiac arrhythmias and headache

Direct Acting Adrenergics

Dr. Evelyn J. Biluk

Word bank

ADRENALINCHLORIDE   ALUPENT   ANXIETY   ARAMINE   BRADYCARDIA   BRETHINE   DOBUTAMINE

DOBUTREX   DOPAMINEHYDROCHLORIDE   EPHEDRINE   INTROPIN   ISOPROTERENOL

ISOXSUPRINEHYDROCHLORIDE   ISUPREL   LEVOPHED   METAPROTERENOLSULFATE   METHOXAMINE

NEO-SYNEPHRINE   NOREPINEPHRINEBITARTRATE   PHENYLEPHRINE   RITODRINE

TERBUTALINESULFATE   VASODILAN   VASOXYL   YUTOPAR

Direct Acting Adrenergics

Dr. Evelyn J. Biluk

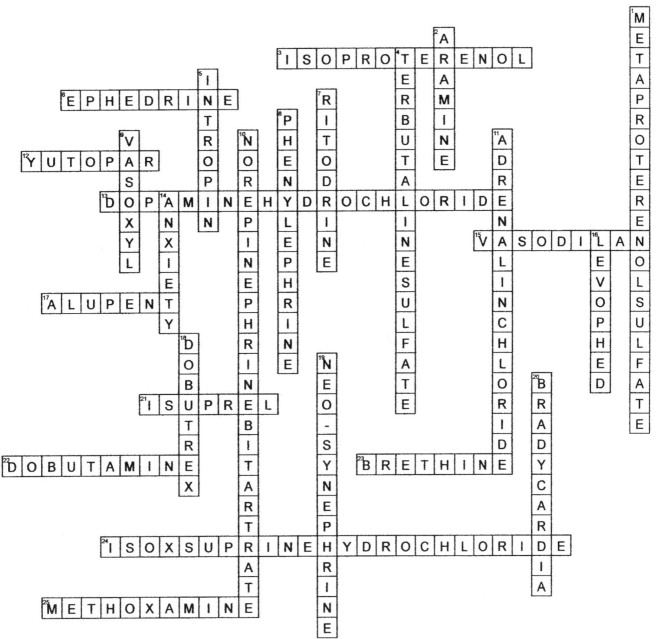

Adrenergic Blocking Agents

Dr. Evelyn J. Biluk

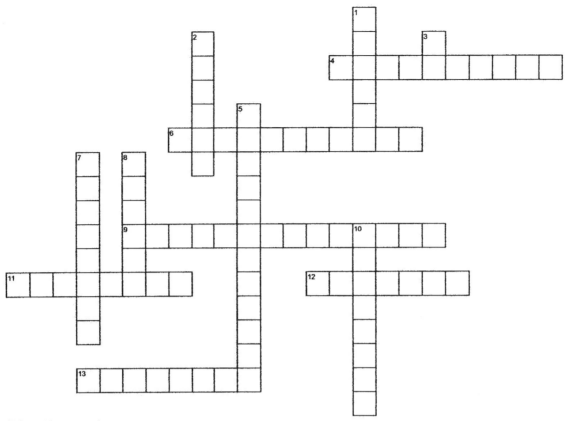

EclipseCrossword.com

Adrenergic Blocking Agents

Dr. Evelyn J. Biluk

Across

4. Ergotamine tartrate is given to adults via _____ or inhalation route

6. Adverse effects of regitine include _____, hypotension, orthostatic hypotension, MI, CV occlusion, arrhythmias, dizziness, weakness, flushing, nausea, vomiting, diarrhea, and nasal stuffiness

9. Used to treat glaucoma and hypertension; Beta-Adrenergic Blocking Agents

11. Ergomar has _____ effects; Contraindicated in pregnant women

12. AKA Ergotamine Tartrate; Alpha-Adrenergic Blocking Agents

13. AKA Phentolamine; Alpha-Adrenergic Blocking Agents

Down

1. Ergotamine tartrate is a drug that is _____ by clients by altering dosage amount

2. Phentolamine blocks _____ receptors thus causing blood vessel dilation

3. Adverse effects of regitine include hypotension, orthostatic hypotension, _____, CV occlusion, tachycardia, arrhythmias, dizziness, weakness, flushing, nausea, vomiting, diarrhea and nasal stuffiness

5. Used for the diagnosis of phenochromocytoma, management of hypertensive episodes in pheochromocytoma, treatment of extravasation from norepinephrine or dopamine hydrochloride, adjunctive therapy in cardiogenic shock or other situations of decreased cardiac output; Alpha-Adrenergic Blocking Agents

7. AKA Timolol Maleate; Beta-Adrenergic Blocking Agents

8. Ergomar has _____ effects

10. Adverse effects of ergomar include _____, nausea, vomiting, numbness, tingling, muscle pain in extremities, pulselessness in legs, precordial pain, transient tachycardia or bradycardia, dependency and abuse

Adrenergic Blocking Agents

Dr. Evelyn J. Biluk

Word bank

ABUSED   ALPHA1   EMETIC   ERGOMAR   ERGOTISM   MI   OXYTOCIC   PHENTOLAMINE

REGITINE   SUBLINGUAL   TACHYCARDIA   TIMOLOLMALEATE   TIMOPTIC

Adrenergic Blocking Agents

Dr. Evelyn J. Biluk

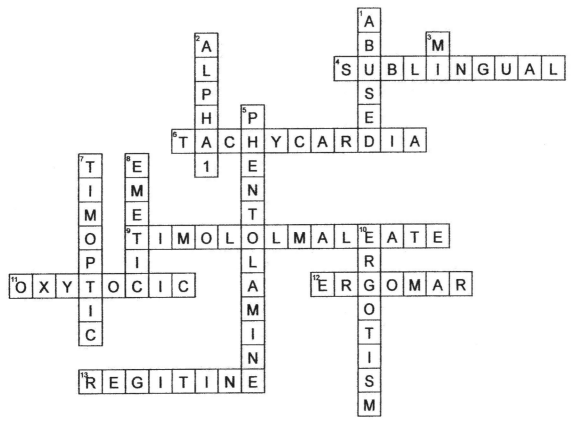

Cholinergics

Dr. Evelyn J. Biluk

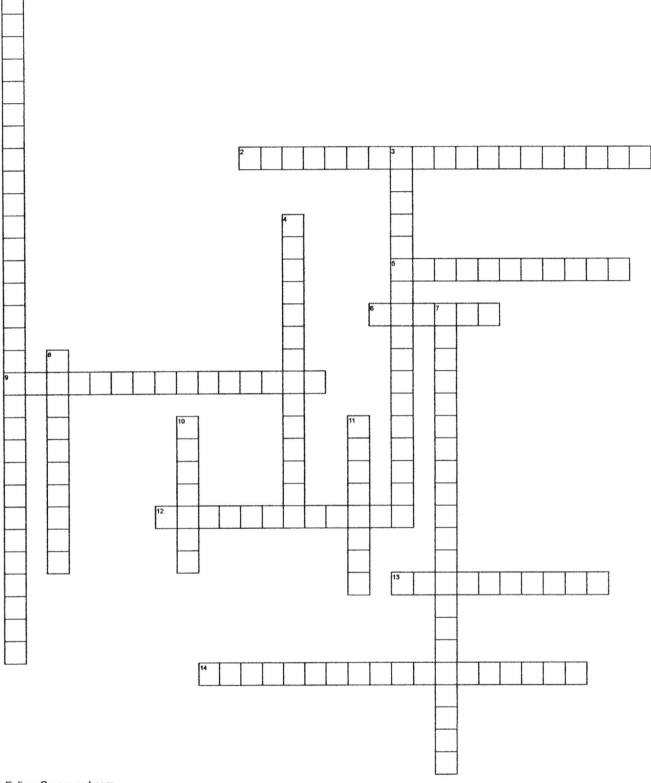

Cholinergics

Dr. Evelyn J. Biluk

Across

2.   Used to treat postoperative urinary retention

5.   Used to treat and diagnose myasthenia gravis, prevent postoperative abdominal distension, treat and prevent postoperative bladder distension, and postoperative reversal of nondepolarizing muscle relaxants

6.   _____ sounds should be monitored in clients taking urecholine to assess for wheezing and bronchospasm

9.   _____ is the antidote for neostigmine

12.   Include miochol and urecholine

13.   AKA Bethanechol Chloride

14.   Adverse effects of miochol include _____, hypotension, bradycardia, bronchospasm, flushing and sweating

Down

1.   Include prostigmin, mestinon and regonol

3.   Adverse effects of acetylcholinesterase inhibitors include _____, nausea, vomiting, cramping, diarrhea, increased salivation, muscle tremor and weakness, dyspnea, bronchospasm, increased bronchial secretions, respiratory depression, hypotension, hypertension, arrhythmias, bradycardia and miosis

4.   Used to treat myasthenia gravis and postoperative reveral of nondepolarizing skeletal muscle relaxants

7.   Used to produce miosis in eye surgery

8.   AKA Neostigmine

10.   AKA Acetylcholine Chloride

11.   AKA Pyridostigmine, Regonol

Cholinergics

Dr. Evelyn J. Biluk

Word bank

ACETYLCHOLINECHLORIDE   ACETYLCHOLINESTERASEINHIBITORS   ATROPINESULFATE

BETHANECHOLCHLORIDE   BREATH   CHOLINERGICCRISIS   CHOLINERGICS   MESTINON   MIOCHOL

NEOSTIGMINE   PROSTIGMIN   PYRIDOSTIGMINE   SYSTEMICABSORPTION   URECHOLINE

Cholinergics

Dr. Evelyn J. Biluk

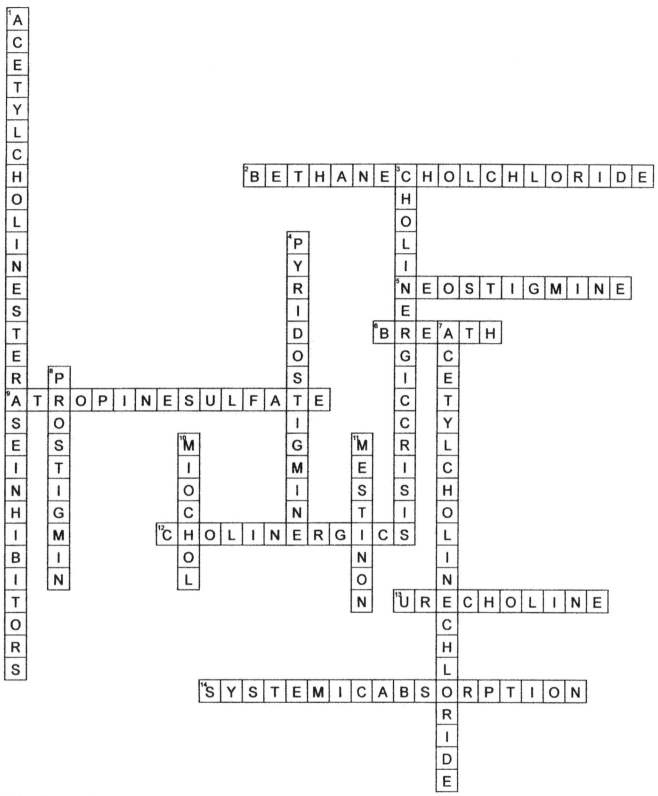

EclipseCrossword.com

Anticholinergics

Dr. Evelyn J. Biluk

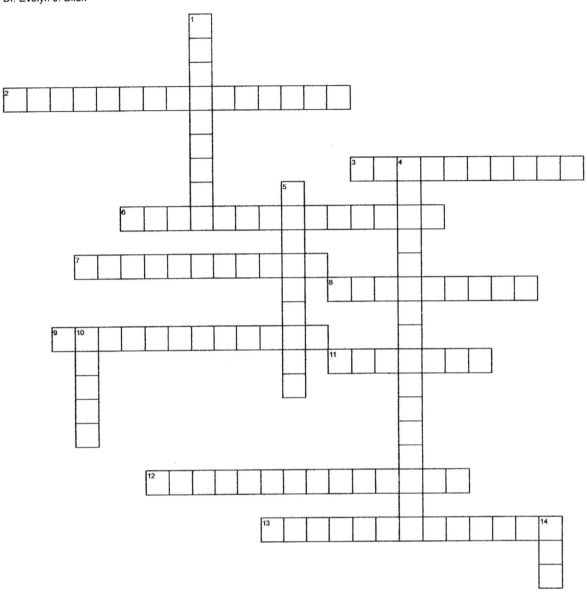

Anticholinergics
Dr. Evelyn J. Biluk

Across

2. Used to produce mydriasis and cycloplegia for eye exams, to treat uveitis, preoperative medication to reduce secretions and bradycardia, treat sinus bradycardia or asystole, hypermotility of GU tract, adjunct in treating asthmatic bronchospasm, GI disorders, antidote for overdoses of parasympathomimetic drugs, prevention of adverse effects when reversing neuromuscular blockade postoperatively with acetylcholine inhibitor and antidote to organophosphate pesticides

3. Cannot give atropine sulfate to patients with _____ gravis

6. Used as preanesthetic medication, adjunct in peptic ulcer disease therapy and reverse neuromuscular blockade

7. Anticholinergic; Used as a preanesthetic medication, midratic and cycloplegic for eye exams, irritable bowel syndrome, diverticulitis and management of postencephalitic parkinsonism

8. _____ foods and fluids should be encouraged for clients on atropine sulfate since it can cause constipation

9. Cannot mix robinul with _____ or alkaline drugs

11. AKA Glycopyrrolate

12. Adverse effects of atropine sulfate include _____, restlessness, hallucinations, headache, dizziness, palpitations, hypertension, hypotension, ventricular tachycardia, blurred vision, photophobia, suppression of sweating, urinary hesitancy and retention, constipation, dry mouth and flushed, dry skin

13. Atropine sulfate is given as a _____ because it causes dry mouth and decreases secretions

Down

1. Cannot give atropine sulfate to patients with _____ hypertrophy

4. _____ include atropine sulfate, scopolamine and robinul

5. Place _____ scop patch behind clients ear the night before trip; Used for prophylaxis of motion sickness

10. Cannot give atropine sulfate to patients with _____ glaucoma

14. Glycopyrrolate has fewer _____ effects than atropine

Anticholinergics

Dr. Evelyn J. Biluk

Word bank

ACUTE   ANTICHOLINERGICS   ATROPINESULFATE   BARBITURATES   CNS   DISORIENTATION

GLYCOPYRROLATE   HIGHFIBER   MYASTHENIA   PREANESTHETIC   PROSTATIC   ROBINUL

SCOPOLAMINE   TRANSDERM

Anticholinergics

Dr. Evelyn J. Biluk

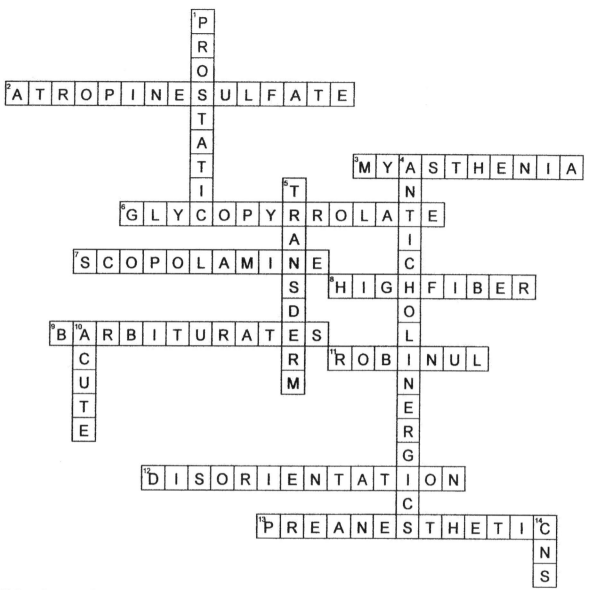

Antiparkinson Agents

Dr. Evelyn J. Biluk

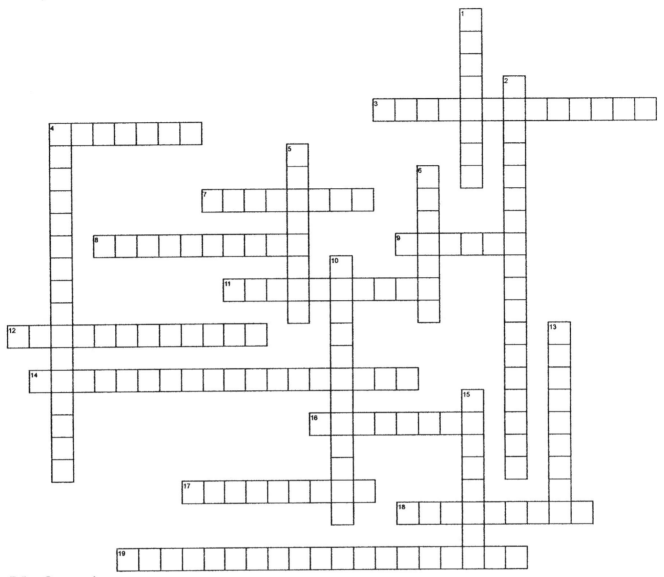

Antiparkinson Agents

Dr. Evelyn J. Biluk

Across

3. Used to treat Parkinson's, female infertility, acromegaly and suppression of postpartum lactation

4. AKA Trihexyphenidyl HCl

7. Adverse effects of artane include _____, constipation, tachycardia, hypotension, dizziness, drowsiness, confusion, decreased bronchial secretions, blurred vision, photophobia, acute glaucoma, urinary retention and suppression of sweating

8. Used to treat idiopathic Parkinson's disease

9. AKA Ropinirole

11. Vitamin B6 (_____) reverses the therapeutic effects of levodopa

12. Artane can cause _____, not diarrhea

14. _____ antagonize the effects of parlodel

16. Congentin has longer lasting _____ effects and muscle relaxation than trihexylphenidyl HCl

17. AKA Benztropine Mesylate

18. AKA Levodopa

19. Used to treat Parkinson's disease, as an adjunct with artane and to control drug-induced extrapyramidal tract symptoms; AKA Congentin

15. Used to treat Parkinson's disease (except drug-induced Parkinson's); AKA Larodopa

Down

1. AKA Bromocriptine

2. Anticholinergic; Antiparkinson agent; Used to treat Parkinson's disease, prevent or control antipsychotic drug-induced extrapyramidal tract symptoms

4. Two categories of antiparkinson agents: _____ and dopaminergic agents

5. Adverse effects of dopaminergic agents include _____, nausea, vomiting, orthostatic hypotension, dizziness, headache, constipation, dry mouth, mydriasis, urinary retention, dark urine, increased BUN/AST/ALT/LDH/bilirubin/alkaline phosphatase, decreased WBCs/hemoglobin/hematocrit, decreased glucose tolerance, blurred vision, muscle twitching, blepharospasm, ataxia, increased hand tremors, disturbed breathing, confusion, anxiety and agitation

6. AKA Carbidopa/Levodopa

10. Two categories of antiparkinson agents: anticholinergics and _____ agents

13. Prevents metabolism of levodopa and allow more of it for transport to the brain; Used to treat Parkinson's disease

Antiparkinson Agents

Dr. Evelyn J. Biluk

Word bank

ANOREXIA   ANTICHOLINERGICS   ARTANEL   BENZTROPINEMESYLATE   BROMOCRIPTINE   CARBIDOPA

CONGENTIN   CONSTIPATION   DOPAMINERGIC   DRYMOUTH   LARODOPAL   LEVODOPA

ORALCONTRACEPTIVES   PARLODEL   PYRIDOXINE   REQUIP   ROPINIROLE   SEDATIVE   SENEMET

TRIHEXYPHENIDYLHCL

Antiparkinson Agents

Dr. Evelyn J. Biluk

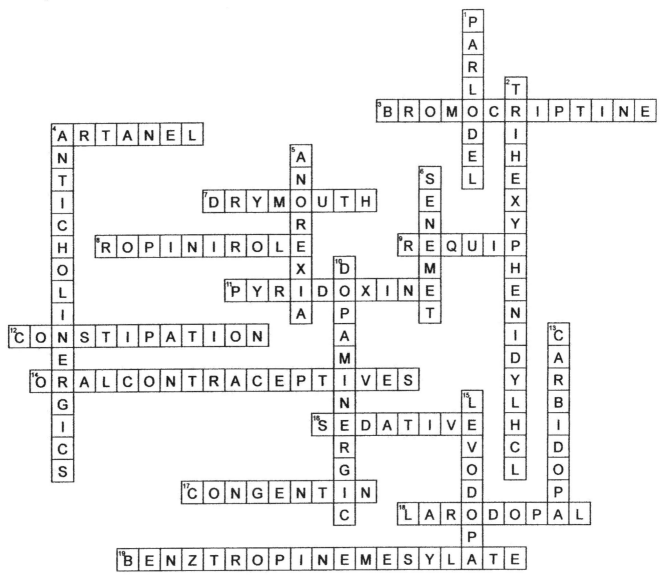

Hypothalamus and Pituitary Gland

Dr. Evelyn J. Biluk

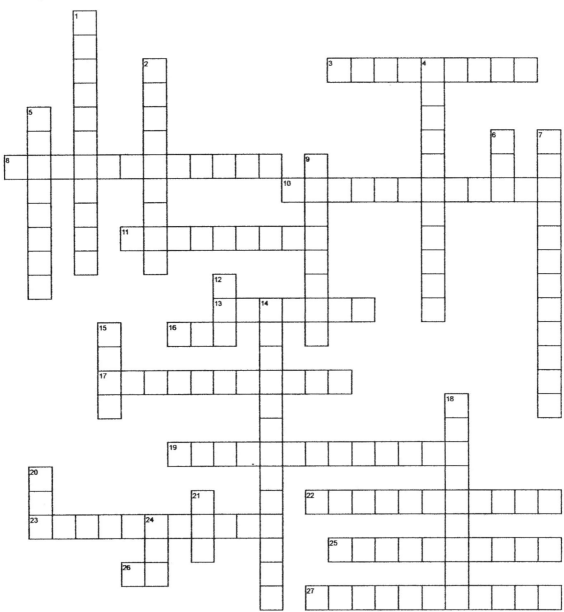

Hypothalamus and Pituitary Gland

Dr. Evelyn J. Biluk

Across

3. _____ gland is also known as the hypophysis
8. Gland that controls the pituitary
10. Stalk that connects the hypothalamus to the pituitary gland
11. _____ glands secrete hormones
13. _____ hormones are derived from cholesterol
16. AKA antidiuretic hormone; Conserve body water by decreasing urine volume
17. Anterior pituitary cells that secrete TSH
19. Anterior pituitary cells that secrete ACTH
22. AKA antiduretic hormone
23. _____ portal system is the flow of blood from hypothalamic capillaries via portal veins to anterior pituitary capillaries
25. _____ hormones suppress the secretion of anterior pituitary hormones
26. AKA luteinizing hormone; In females, stimulates estrogen and progesterone secretion
27. Anterior pituitary cells that secrete PRL

Down

1. AKA NO; A hormone and neurotransmitter
2. _____ hormones stimulate the secretion of anterior pituitary hormones
4. _____ growth factors (AKA IGFs); Cause cells to grow and multiply by increasing the uptake of amino acids during protein synthesis
5. AKA OT; Stimulates uterus to contract during childbirth
6. AKA prolactin; Promotes milk secretion by mammary glands
7. Anterior pituitary cells that secrete hGH
9. _____ pituitary (AKA adenohypophysis)
12. AKA follicle stimulating hormone; In females, stimulates oocyte development and estrogen *secretion by the ovaries*
14. Study of endocrine glands and the diagnosis and treatment of endocrine system disorders
15. AKA corticotropin; Stimulates glucocorticoid secretion by adrenal cortex
18. _____ pituitary (AKA neurohypophysis)
20. AKA melanocyte stimulating hormone; Function unknown
21. AKA thyrotropin; Stimulates synthesis and secretion of thyroid hormones

24. AKA human growth hormone; Stimulates tissues like muscle and bone to synthesize and secrete IGFs

Hypothalamus and Pituitary Gland

Dr. Evelyn J. Biluk

Word bank

ACTH   ADH   ANTERIOR   CORTICOTROPHS   ENDOCRINE   ENDOCRINOLOGY   FSH   HGH

HYPOPHYSEAL   HYPOTHALAMUS   INFUNDIBULUM   INHIBITING   INSULINLIKE   LACTOTROPHS   LH

MSH   NITRICOXIDE   OXYTOCIN   PITUITARY   POSTERIOR   PRL   RELEASING   SOMATOTROPHS

STEROID   THYROTROPHS   TSH   VASOPRESSIN

Hypothalamus and Pituitary Gland

Dr. Evelyn J. Biluk

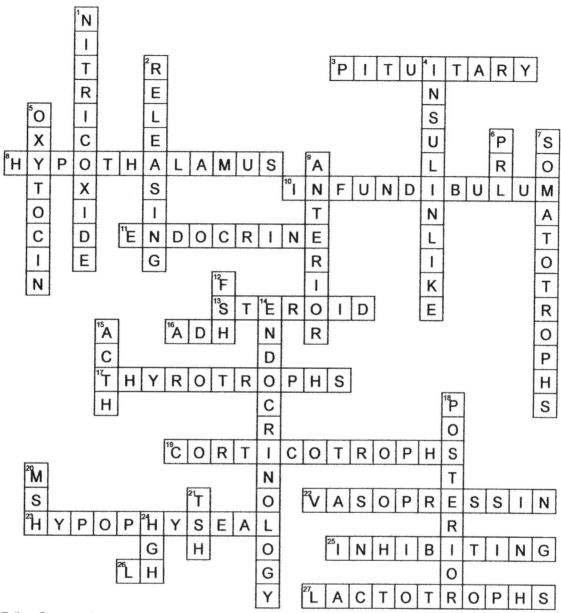

EclipseCrossword.com

Endocrine System: Thyroid, Parathyroid and Adrenal Glands

Dr. Evelyn J. Biluk

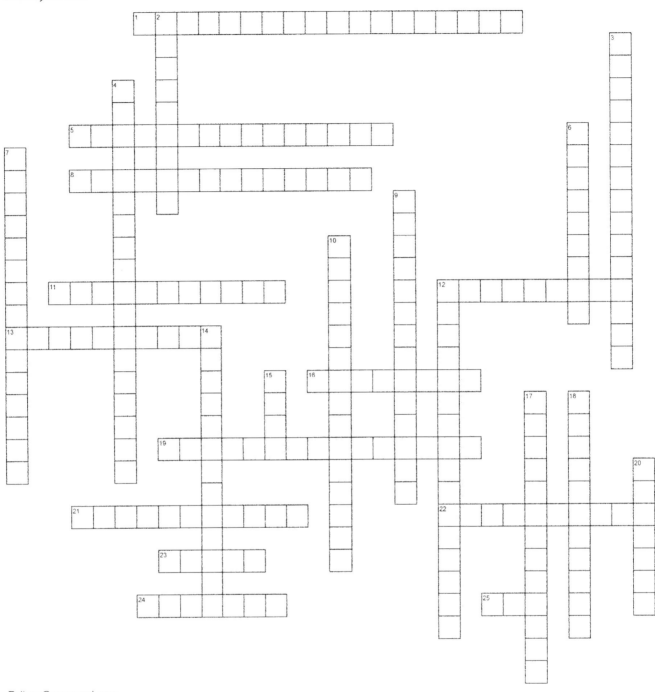

Endocrine System: Thyroid, Parathyroid and Adrenal Glands

Dr. Evelyn J. Biluk

Across

1. AKA PTH; Increases blood calcium levels
5. Outer zone of adrenal cortex
8. Central portion of adrenal glands
11. Main mineralocorticoid hormone
12. AKA T4
13. AKA CT; Lowers blood calcium levels
16. Main glucocorticoid hormone
19. Middle zone of adrenal cortex
21. Adrenal medulla hormone that enhances the sympathetic nervous system during stress
22. Renin-angiotensin-aldosterone pathway; Controls the secretion of aldosterone
23. _____ cells produce PTH
24. _____ glands lies superior to each kidney
25. Basal metabolic rate; Rate of oxygen consumption *under standard conditions (awake, at rest, fasting)*

Down

2. Adrenal cortex hormones that assist in axillary and pubic hair in both males and females
3. Conversion of a substance other than glycogen or another monosaccharide into glucose
4. Adrenal cortex hormones that increase sodium and water levels in the blood and decrease potassium levels in the blood
6. Glucocorticoids stimulate _____, the breakdown of triglycerides and release of fatty acids from adipose tissue into the blood
7. Inner zone of adrenal cortex
9. _____ cells produce calcitonin
10. Adrenal cortex hormones that increase protein breakdown, provide resistance to stress, dampen inflammation and depress the immune responses
12. AKA T3
14. AKA noradrenalin; Similar function to adrenalin (epinephrine)
15. Main androgen hormone
17. Outer region of adrenal glands
18. _____ gland is located on the posterior surface of the lateral lobes of the thyroid gland
20. _____ gland is located just inferior to the larynx

Endocrine System: Thyroid, Parathyroid and Adrenal Glands

Dr. Evelyn J. Biluk

Word bank

ADRENAL   ADRENALCORTEX   ADRENALMEDULLA   ALDOSTERONE   ANDROGENS   BMR

CALCITONIN   CHIEF   CORTISOL   DHEA   EPINEPHRINE   GLUCOCORTICOIDS   GLUCONEOGENESIS

LIPOLYSIS   MINERALOCORTICOIDS   NORPINEPHRINE   PARAFOLLICULAR   PARATHYROID

PARATHYROIDHORMONE   RAAPATHWAY   THYROID   THYROXINE   TRIIODOTHYRONINE

ZONAFASCICULATA   ZONAGLOMERULOSA   ZONARETICULARIS

Endocrine System: Thyroid, Parathyroid and Adrenal Glands

Dr. Evelyn J. Biluk

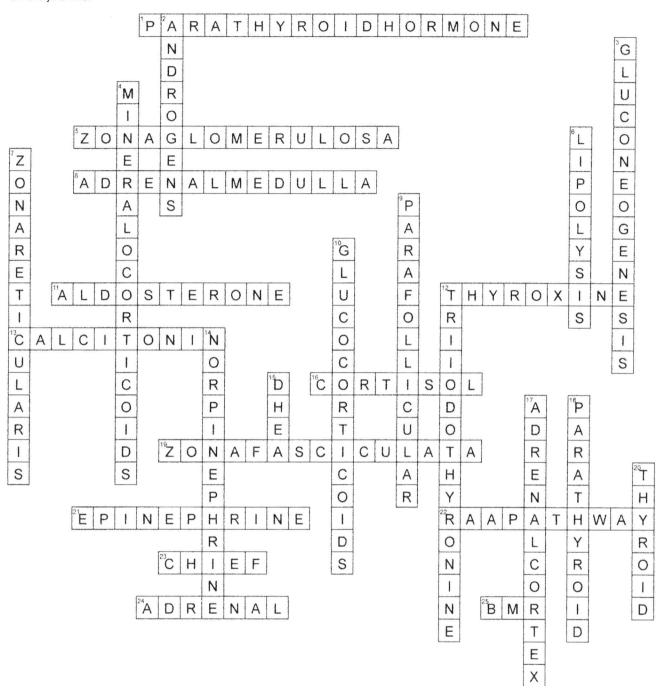

EclipseCrossword.com

Endocrine System: Pancreas, Ovaries, Testes and Pineal Gland

Dr. Evelyn J. Biluk

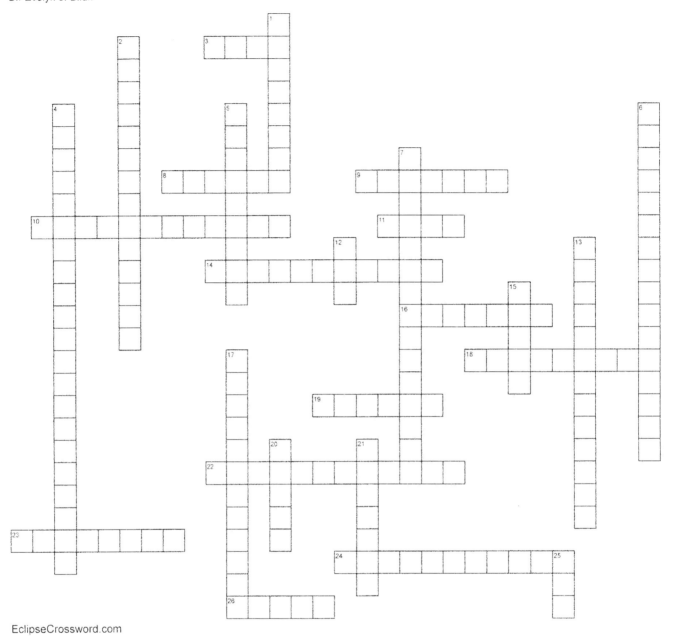

Endocrine System: Pancreas, Ovaries, Testes and Pineal Gland

Dr. Evelyn J. Biluk

Across

3. _____ cells also known as B cells; Secrete insulin

8. _____ are organs that produce gametes

9. Peptide hormone that increases the flexibility of the pubic symphysis during pregnancy; Also dilates the cervix during labor and delivery

10. Male hormone that regulates spermatogenesis, stimulates the descent of the testes and promotes the development and maintenance of male secondary sex characteristics

11. AKA adrenocorticotropic hormone; Also stimulates the secretion of insulin

14. _____ is an endocrine gland attached the roof of the 3rd ventricle

16. Paired oval bodies in the female pelvic cavity

18. _____ and progesterone regulate the female reproductive cycle, regulate oogenesis, maintain pregnancy, prepare the mammary glands for lactation and promote the development and maintenance of female secondary sex characteristics

19. Oval glands that lie in the male scrotum

22. Insulin speeds up the conversion of glucose into glycogen in a process known as _____

23. Male sex hormone

24. Insulin speeds up the synthesis of fatty acids in a process known as _____

26. _____ or A cells secrete glucagon

20. Cells arranged in clusters in the pancreas that produce digestive enzymes for the GI tract

21. In females and males, this hormone inhibits the secretion of follicle stimulating hormone from the anterior pituitary

25. AKA seasonal affective disorder; Type of depression affecting people during winter

Down

1. An endocrine gland and an exocrine gland

2. Glucagon acts on liver cells to stimulate this process; The conversion of glycogen into glucose

4. F cells in the pancreas secrete _____

5. Hormone produced by the pineal gland; Contributes to the setting of the body's biological clock

6. AKA Islets of Langerhans; Cluster of endocrine tissue found in the pancreas

7. Glucagon stimulates the liver cells to promote the formation of glucose from lactic acid and amino acids in a process called _____

12. AKA human growth hormone; Responsible for stimulating the secretion of insulin

13. _____ (high blood glucose) stimulates the beta cells to secrete insulin

15. _____ cells AKA D cells; Produce somatostatin

17. _____ (low blood glucose) stimulates alpha cells to secrete glucagon

Endocrine System: Pancreas, Ovaries, Testes and Pineal Gland

Dr. Evelyn J. Biluk

Word bank

ACINI   ACTH   ALPHA   ANDROGEN   BETA   DELTA   ESTROGENS   GLUCONEOGENESIS

GLYCOGENESIS   GLYCOGENOLYSIS   GONADS   HGH   HYPERGLYCEMIA   HYPOGLYCEMIA   INHIBIN

LIPOGENESIS   MELATONIN   OVARIES   PANCREAS   PANCREATICISLETS

PANCREATICPOLYPEPTIDE   PINEALGLAND   RELAXIN   SAD   TESTES   TESTOSTERONE

Endocrine System: Pancreas, Ovaries, Testes and Pineal Gland

Dr. Evelyn J. Biluk

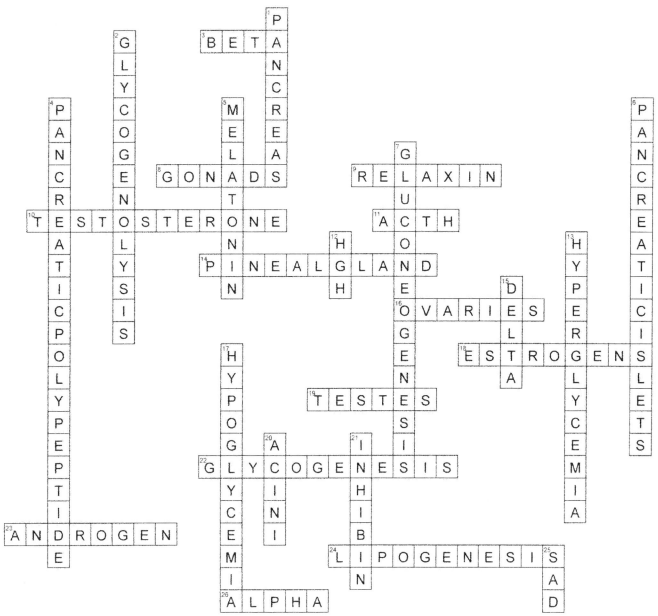

Endocrine System: Thymus and Other Endocrine Tissues

Dr. Evelyn J. Biluk

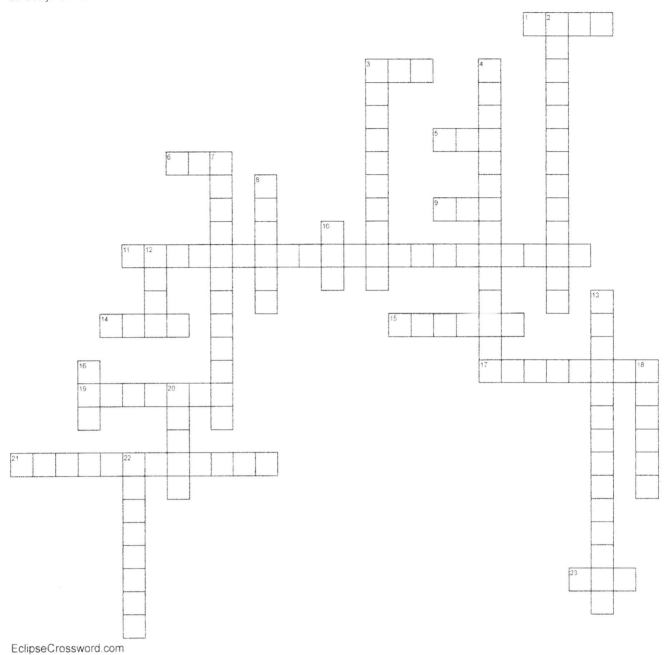

Endocrine System: Thymus and Other Endocrine Tissues

Dr. Evelyn J. Biluk

Across

1. Also known as transforming growth factors; Subtypes include alpha and beta

3. AKA cholecystokinin; Stimulates the secretion of pancreatic juice, regulates bile release from the gallbladder and brings about a feeling of fullness after eating

5. Also known as human chorionic somatomammotropin; Stimulates the development of mammary glands for lactation

6. Also known as atrial natriuretic peptide; Decreases BP

9. AKA human chorionic gonadotropin; Stimulates corpus luteum to produce estrogens and progesterone to maintain pregnancy

11. AKA EGF; Stimulates the proliferation of epithelial cells, fibroblasts, neurons, and astrocytes; Suppresses some cancer cells and secretion of gastric juice

14. AKA tumor angiogenesis factors; Stimulate the growth of new capillaries, organ regeneration and wound healing

15. Adipose tissue hormone; Suppresses appetite and may increase the activity of FSH and LH

17. GI tract hormone that stimulates the secretion of pancreatic juice and bile

19. GI tract hormone that promotes the secretion of gastric juice and increases stomach movements

21. Eicosanoid molecules; Stimulate chemotaxis of WBCs and mediates inflammation

23. AKA glucose-dependent insulinotropic peptide; Stimulates the release of insulin by the beta cells

12. AKA platelet-derived growth factor; Stimulates the proliferation of neuroglia, smooth muscle fibers and fibroblasts

13. AKA EPO; Increases the rate of RBC formation

16. Also known as fibroblast growth factor; Stimulates the proliferation of many cells derived from mesoderm

18. Drugs that inhibit prostaglandin synthesis; Reduce fever, pain, and inflammation

20. Kidney hormone; Raises BP via vasoconstriction and secretion of aldosterone

22. _____, thymic humoral factor, thymic factor and thymopoietin are all hormones that promote the maturation of T cells

Down

2. Recently discovered hormones that play an important role in tissue development, growth and repair

3. Kidney hormone; Aids in the absorption of dietary calcium and phosphorus

4. Eicosanoid molecules; Alter smooth muscle contraction, glandular secretions, blood flow, reproductive processes, platelet function, respiraton and nerve impulse transmission

7. Estrogens and _____ maintain pregnancy and help prepare mammary glands to secrete milk

8. Endocrine gland located behind the sternum between the lungs

10. Also known as nerve growth factor; Stimulates the growth of ganglia in the embryo; Maintains the SNS; Stimulates the hypertrophy and differentiation of neurons

Endocrine System: Thymus and Other Endocrine Tissues

Dr. Evelyn J. Biluk

Word bank

ANP   CALCITRIOL   CCK   EPIDERMALGROWTHFACTOR   ERYTHROPOIETIN   FGF   GASTRIN   GIP

GROWTHFACTORS   HCG   HCS   LEPTIN   LEUKOTRIENES   NGF   NSAIDS   PDGF

PROGESTERONE   PROSTAGLANDINS   RENIN   SECRETIN   TAFS   TGFS   THYMOSIN   THYMUS

Endocrine System: Thymus and Other Endocrine Tissues

Dr. Evelyn J. Biluk

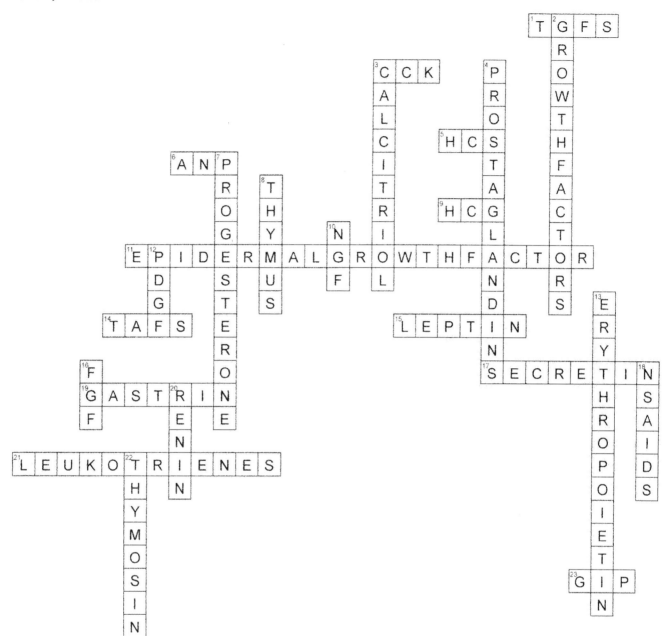

EclipseCrossword.com

Antidiabetic Agents

Dr. Evelyn J. Biluk

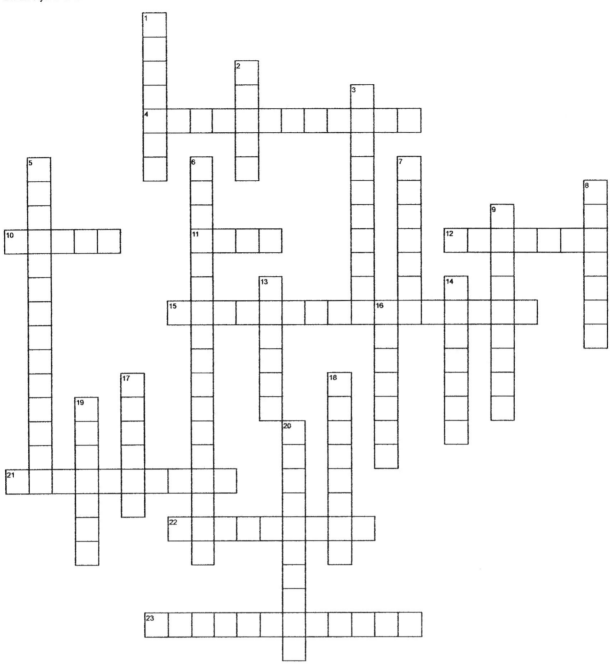

Antidiabetic Agents

Dr. Evelyn J. Biluk

Across

4. AKA insulin zinc, suspension

10. Clients allegic to _____ cannot be taken with orinase

11. Insulin should be at _____ temperature before injecting to decrease occurrence of lipodystrophy

12. AKA Tolbutamide; Used for Type II diabetes (not controlled by diet and exercise); Used with insulin in Type II diabetic when neither insulin nor oral hypoglycemic agents work well alone

15. AKA insulin (zinc suspension, prompt)

21. Oral antidiabetic agents can only work when the client has _____ insulin

22. AKA Diabeta, Glyburide; Oral sulfonylureas; Duration of action 10-24 hours

23. Adverse effects of insulin include allergic reaction (local or systemic), hypoglycemia and _____

Down

1. AKA Acetohexamide; Oral sulfonylureas; Duration of action 12-24 hours

2. _____ appearance is associated with regular insulin

3. AKA Metformin; Oral biguanides; Duration of action 10-16 hours

5. AKA rapid acting insulin injection

6. AKA long acting, insulin zinc suspension, extended

7. AKA Troglitazone; Oral alpha-glucosidose inhibitor; Peak action is 2 to 3 hours

8. AKA Acarbose; Oral alpha-glucosidase inhibitor; Peak action is 1 hour

9. AKA Chlorpropamide; Oral Sulfonylureas; Duraiton of action 40-60 hours

13. _____ appearance is associated with semilente insulin, NPH insulin, lente insulin and ultralente insulin

14. Insulin lispro; A synthetic insulin with a faster onset and shorter duration of action than human insulin

16. Antidiabetic agent; Used for Type I diabetic clients; Used for Type II diabetics not controlled with oral hypoglycemic agents, diet and exercise; Used for Type II diabetics undergoing stressful situations (infection or surgery); Used for pregnant diabetic women; Used for emergency management of diabetic coma

17. AKA Miglitol; Oral alpha-glucosidose inhibitor; Peak action is 2 to 3 hours

18. _____ increases glucose use in the body

19. _____ combined with an oral hypoglycemic agent can trigger a hypoglycemic reaction

20. AKA intermediate acting, isophane insulin injection

Antidiabetic Agents

Dr. Evelyn J. Biluk

Word bank

ALCOHOL   CLEAR   CLOUDY   DIABINASE   DYMELOR   ENDOGENOUS   EXERCISE   GLUCOPHAGE

GLYSET   HUMALOG   INSULIN   KETOACIDOSIS   LENTEINSULIN   MICRONASE   NPHINSULIN

ORINASE   PRECOSE   REGULARINSULIN   REZULIN   ROOM   SEMILENTEINSULIN   SULFA

ULTRALENTEINSULIN

Antidiabetic Agents

Dr. Evelyn J. Biluk

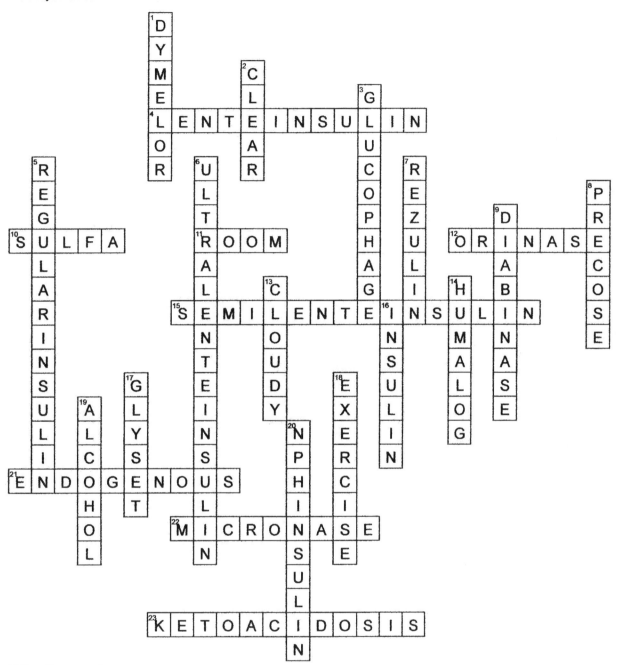

Pituitary Hormones

Dr. Evelyn J. Biluk

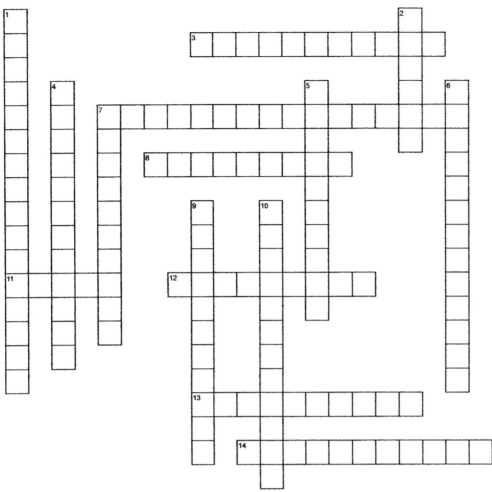

Pituitary Hormones

Dr. Evelyn J. Biluk

Across

3. Used as a diagnostic test to diagnose adrenal insufficiency

7. Adverse effects of ADH include _____, anaphylaxis, water intoxication, hyponatremia, nausea, diarrhea, cramping, hypertension, nasal irritation and headache

8. AKA Vasopressin; ADH (antidiuretic hormone)

11. AKA Desmopressin

12. AKA Cosyntropin; Synthetic corticotropin

13. Used for replacement therapy in children with growth retardation due to a lack of somatotropin

14. Vasopressin is a _____ for ADH hormone

Down

1. _____ is an adverse effect of cortrosyn if given over a period of time

2. AKA Lypressin

4. Desmopressin can be given PO, SC, IV or _____

5. _____ is reduced by drinking a glass of water when taking vasopressin

6. Adverse effects of humatropel include _____, pain at injection site, myalgia, headache, hypercalciuria and allergic reactions

7. AKA Somatropin

9. Used for replacement therapy for diabetes insipidus

10. DDVAP must be _____

Pituitary Hormones

Dr. Evelyn J. Biluk

Word bank

CORTROSYN   COSYNTROPIN   CUSHINGSSYNDROME   DDAVP   DIAPID   GIDISTRESS

HUMATROPEL   HYPERGLYCEMIA   HYPERSENSITIVITY   INTRANASALLY   PITRESSIN   REFRIGERATED

REPLACEMENT   SOMATROPIN   VASOPRESSIN

Pituitary Hormones

Dr. Evelyn J. Biluk

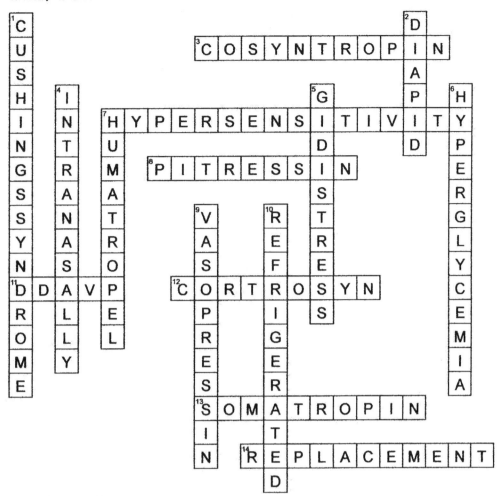

EclipseCrossword.com

Thyroid Hormones

Dr. Evelyn J. Biluk

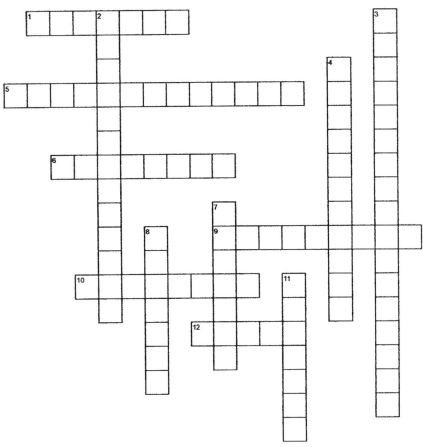

Thyroid Hormones

Dr. Evelyn J. Biluk

Across

1.   AKA Thyroglobulin

5.   Used for dessicated thyroid; AKA Proloid

6.   AKA Liotrex

9.   AKA Levothyroxine

10. Adverse effects of synthroid include _____, headache, nervousness, irritability, palpitations, increased angina, weight loss, nausea, vomiting, menstrual irregularities, allergic skin reaction and heat intolerance

12. Protect levothyroxine from _____

Down

2.   Used to replace or substitute diminished or absent thyroid fuction due to thyroid disease or thyroidectomy

3.   Used for dessicated thyroid; AKA Cytomel

4.   A nurse should check the patient for _____ via checking the pulse before administration of levothyroxine

7.   Patients on synthroid should avoid _____ use

8.   Used for dessicated thyroid; AKA Thyrolar

11. AKA Liothyronine Sodium

Thyroid Hormones

Dr. Evelyn J. Biluk

Word bank

ASPIRIN   CYTOMEL   INSOMNIA   LEVOTHYROXINE   LIGHT   LIOTHYRONINSODIUM   LIOTREX
PROLOID   SYNTHROID   TACHYCARDIA   THYROGLOBULIN   THYROLAR

Thyroid Hormones

Dr. Evelyn J. Biluk

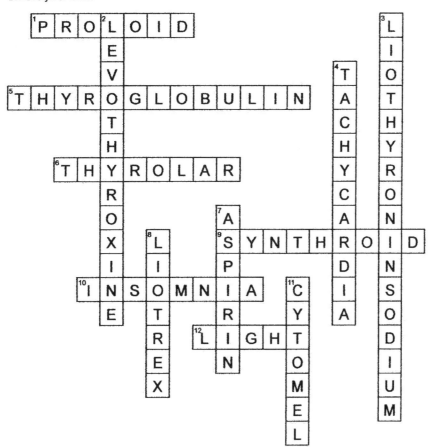

EclipseCrossword.com

Thyroid Antagonists

Dr. Evelyn J. Biluk

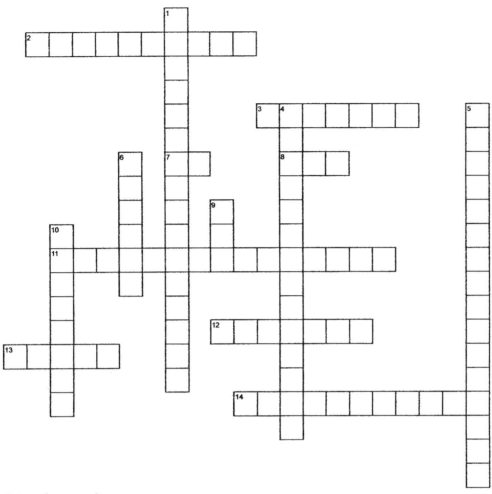

Thyroid Antagonists

Dr. Evelyn J. Biluk

Across

2. _____ is an adverse effect of iodines

3. PTU prevents the synthesis of _____ hormones

7. PTU partially prevents the peripheral conversion of _____ to T3

8. AKA Propylthiouracil

11. Signs of _____ include fever, chills and sore throat

12. Low doses necessary for thyroid function; High doses inhibit thyroid function; Used to treat hyperthyroidism and thyroid cancer

13. Signs of agranulocytosis require _____ work immediately

14. Used to management hyperthyroidism; Ten times more potent than PTU; Given once daily

Down

1. Used to manage hyperthyroidism

4. Risk of _____ is less with methimazole

5. Adverse effects of thyroid antagonists include _____, hypothyroidism, agranulocytosis, bleeding, nausea, vomiting, loss of taste, rash, urticaria, skin pigmentation, jaundice, hepatitis and nephritis

6. Signs of agranulocytosis require a _____ culture

9. PTU response occurs _____ to three weeks after starting the drug

10. AKA Methimazole

Thyroid Antagonists

Dr. Evelyn J. Biluk

Word bank

AGRANULOCYTOSIS   BLOOD   GIDISTRESS   HEPATOTOXICITY   IODINES   METHIMAZOLE

PROPYLTHIOURACIL   PTU   T4   TAPAZOLE   THROAT   THROMBOCYTOPENIA   THYROID   TWO

Thyroid Antagonists

Dr. Evelyn J. Biluk

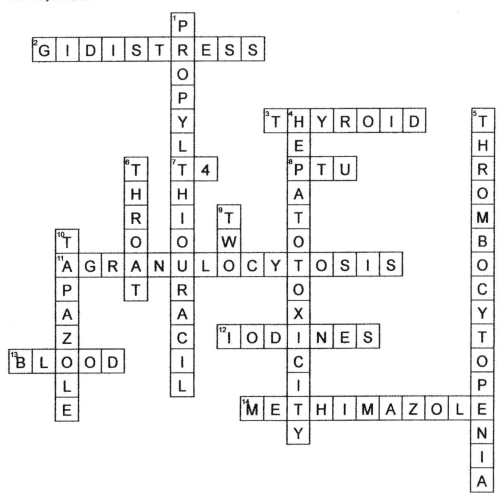

EclipseCrossword.com

Women's Health Agents

Dr. Evelyn J. Biluk

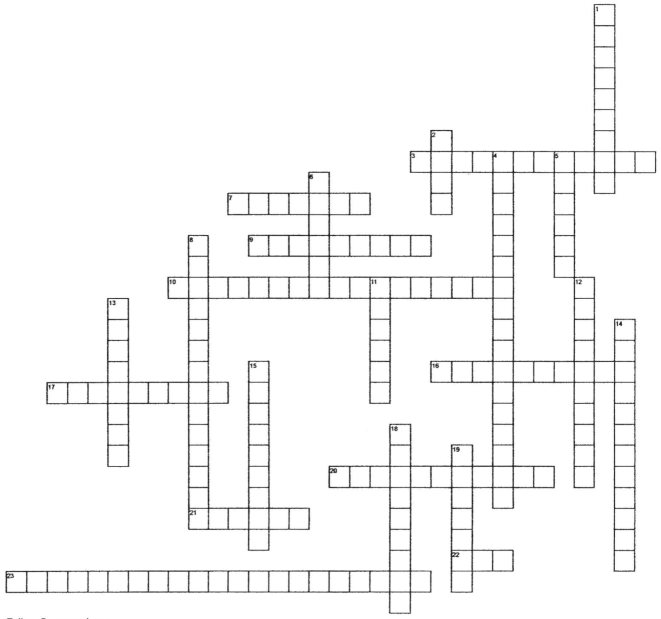

Women's Health Agents

Dr. Evelyn J. Biluk

Across

3. Used for amenorrhea, abnormal uterine bleeding, endometrial cancer and prevention of conception

7. AKA Medroxyprogesterone

9. AKA Hydroxyprogesterone

10. Used for infertility and induces ovulation

16. AKA Evista; Used to prevent postmenopausal osteoporosis

17. AKA Novadex; Used to prevent and treat breast cancer

20. _____ are given IM; Fertility Agents; AKA Pergonal

21. AKA Tiludronate; Used to prevent osteoporosis and Paget's disease

22. AKA Chorionic Gonadotropin

23. _____ is given IM; Also known as A.P.L.; Fertility Agents

Down

1. Estrogen-progestin combinations suppress _____ by preventing release of FSH and LH

2. _____ contraceptives include estrogen-progestin combinations and progestin-only preparations

4. _____ combinations are more effective than progestin-only preparations

5. _____ and Novadex are selective estrogen receptor modulators

6. AKA Megesterolacetate

8. Adverse effects of fertility agents include _____, headache, tachycardia, nausea, vomiting, constipation, anxiety, DVT, breast pain and diplopia

11. AKA Clomiphene Citrate

12. Estrogen-progestin combinations are used for _____ of pregnancy, amenorrhea, functional bleeding and endometriosis

13. AKA Menotropins

14. In parenteral administration, adverse effects of progestin include _____ bleeding, spotting, dysmenorrhea, breast tenderness, headache, dizziness, edema, thromboembolism, hypertension, nausea, vomiting, bloating, weight gain, jaundice, rash, hirsutism, acne, oily skin and vision changes

15. Progestin-only preparations are known as _____

18. AKA Progesterone

19. AKA Alendronate; Use to prevent and treat osteoporosis and Paget's disease

Women's Health Agents

Dr. Evelyn J. Biluk

Word bank

APL   BREAKTHROUGH   CHORIONICGONADOTROPIN   CLOMID   CLOMIPHENECITRATE   DELALUTIN
ESTROGENPROGESTIN   EVISTA   FOSAMAX   MEGACE   MENOTROPINS   MINIPILLS
MULTIPLEBIRTHS   ORAL   OVULATION   PERGONAL   PREVENTION   PROGESTERONE   PROGESTIN
PROVERA   RALOXIFENE   SKELID   TAMOXIFEN

Women's Health Agents

Dr. Evelyn J. Biluk

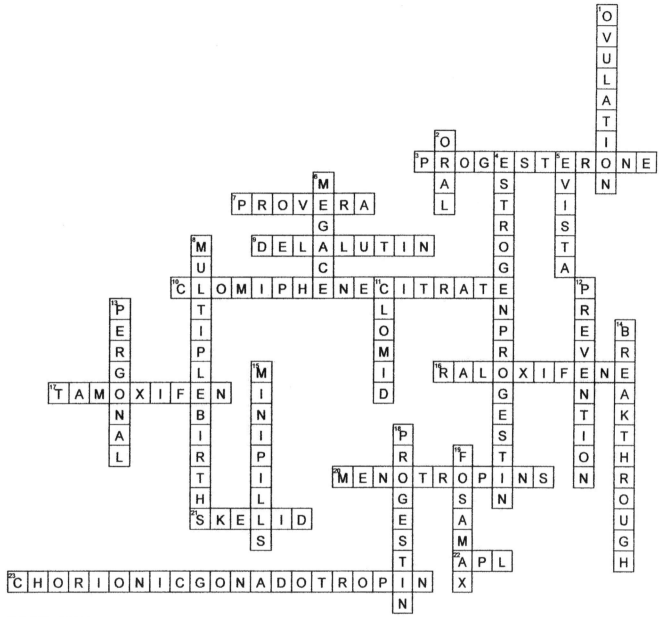

Men's Health Agents

Dr. Evelyn J. Biluk

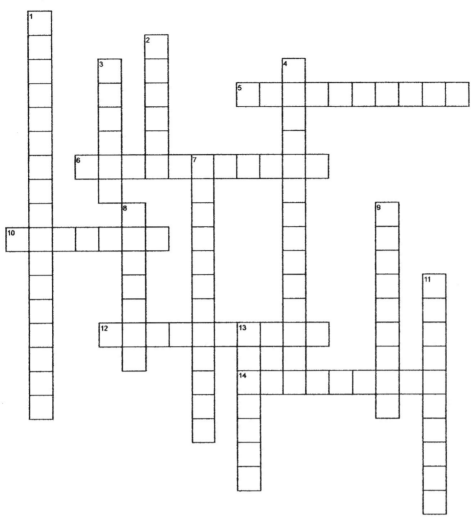

Men's Health Agents

Dr. Evelyn J. Biluk

Across

5.   AKA Fluoxymesterone

6.   Used to treat BPH

10.   AKA Vardenafil

12.   AKA Levitra; Used to treat male erectile dysfunction

14.   AKA Danazol

Down

1.   _____ inhibitors include viagra, cialis and levitra

2.   AKA Sildenafil

3.   AKA Tadalafil

4.   Adverse effects of androgens include _____, headaches, nausea, vomiting, constipation, diarrhea, acne, gynecomastia, priapism, depression, jaundice and bleeding

7.   Androgen; Primarily used for replacement therapy

8.   AKA Finasteride; Androgen inhibitor

9.   Used to treat male erectile dysfunction

11.   Used to treat male erectile dysfunction; AKA Viagra

13.   AKA Methytestosterone

Men's Health Agents

Dr. Evelyn J. Biluk

Word bank

ANDROID   CIALIS   DANOCRINE   FINASTERIDE   FLUIDRETENTION   HALOTESTIN   LEVITRA

PHOSPHODIESTERASE   PROSCAR   SILDENAFIL   TADALAFIL   TESTOSTERONE   VARDENAFIL

VIAGRA

Men's Health Agents

Dr. Evelyn J. Biluk

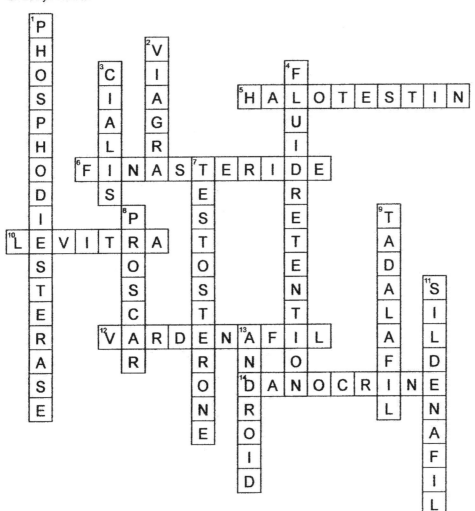

Oxytocics

Dr. Evelyn J. Biluk

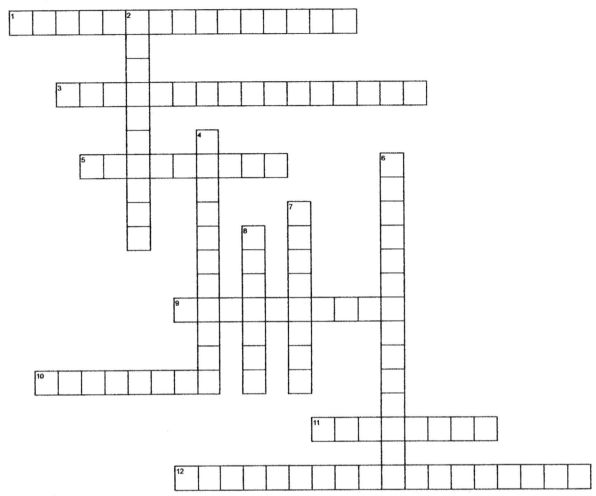

Oxytocics

Dr. Evelyn J. Biluk

Across

1. Oxytocin is administered _____ after delivery of the placenta

3. AKA Methergine; Used as prophylaxis after the delivery of the placenta

5. AKA Ergonovine

9. Used to control late postpartum bleeding, treat and prevent postpartum and postabortion bleeding

10. Methergine cannot be administered before delivery of the _____

11. Oxytocin infusion should be administered on an _____ pump

12. _____, bradycardia, nausea, vomiting and diarrhea are all adverse effects of ergotrate

Down

2. AKA Methylergonovine

4. Adverse effects of pitocin in the fetus include _____, hypoxia, intracranial hemorrhage, death and anaphylactic reactions

6. Adverse effects of pitocin include _____, water intoxication, hypotension, postpartum hemorrhage, PVCs, cardiac arrhythmias, nausea, vomiting, hypertension, cardiovascular collapse

7. Used to induce labor, control postpartum bleeding, treatment of incomplete abortion and stimulate breast milk injection

8. AKA Oxytocin

Oxytocics

Dr. Evelyn J. Biluk

Word bank

BRADYCARDIA   ERGONOVINE   ERGOTRATE   INFUSION   INTRAMUSCULARLY   METHERGINE

METHYLERGONOVINE   OXYTOCIN   PITOCIN   PLACENTA   SEVEREHYPERTENSION   UTERINERUPTURE

Oxytocics

Dr. Evelyn J. Biluk

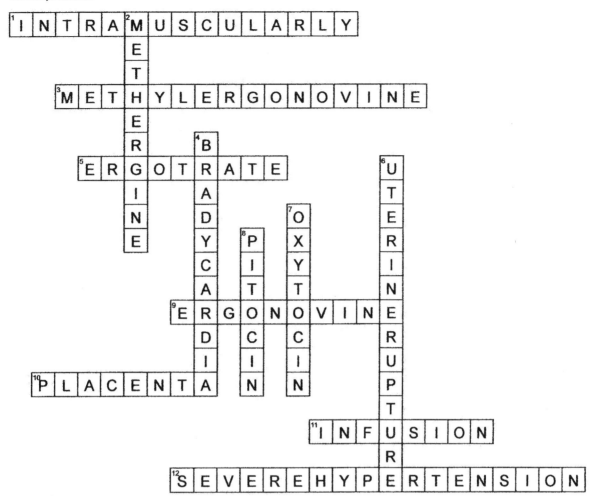

Mydriatics and Cycloplegics

Dr. Evelyn J. Biluk

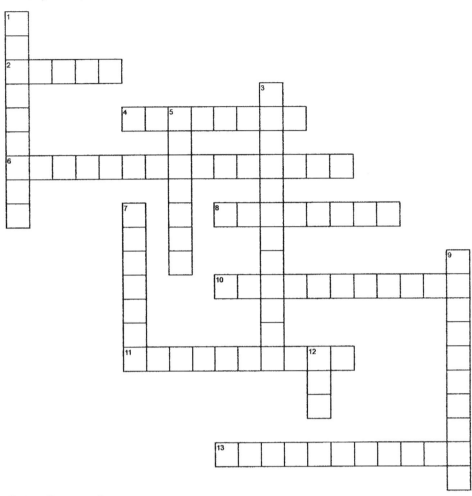

Mydriatics and Cycloplegics

Dr. Evelyn J. Biluk

Across

2. Clients should not _____ until the effects of atropine have worn off

4. AKA Apraclonidine; A sympathomimetic agent

6. _____ agents work in a manner similar to atropine on the sympathetic nervous system

8. AKA Cyclopentolate; Also classified as a sympathomimetic drug

10. Atropine can raise _____ pressure; Clients with glaucoma have increased _____ pressure -- a further increase could lead to acute crisis and blindness

11. _____ can be used by patients to reduce photophobia

13. Adverse effects of atropine include _____, reduced lacrimation, impaired distant vision, increased intraocular pressure, eye pain and blurred vision

Down

1. Dilation of the pupil

3. Applying pressure to the _____ will reduce systemic effects related to the use of atropine

5. AKA Dipivefrin; Classified as a sympathomimetic agent

7. Atropine is used to treat _____

9. _____ tears are used for reduced lacrimation

12. Atropine is used to facilitate _____ exams

Mydriatics and Cycloplegics

Dr. Evelyn J. Biluk

Word bank

ARTIFICIAL   CYCLOGYL   DRIVE   EYE   INNERCANTHUS   INTRAOCULAR   IOPIDINE   MYDRIASIS
PHOTOPHOBIA   PROPINE   SUNGLASSES   SYMPATHOMIMETIC   UVEITIS

Mydriatics and Cycloplegics

Dr. Evelyn J. Biluk

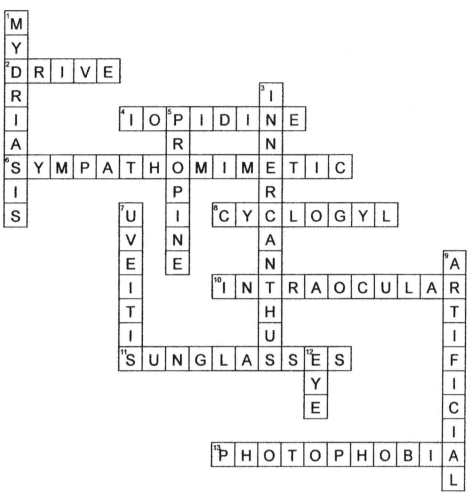

Miotics

Dr. Evelyn J. Biluk

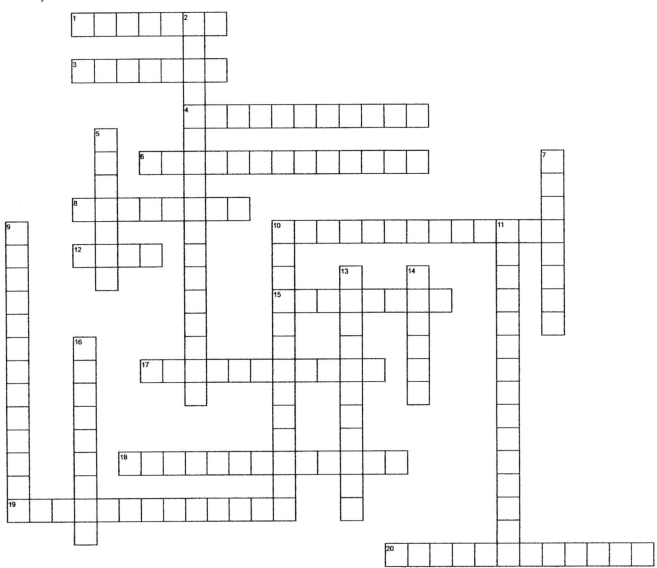

Miotics

Dr. Evelyn J. Biluk

Across

1. AKA Dorzolamide

3. AKA Acetylcholine

4. AKA Pilocar

6. AKA Pilocar or Pilocarpine; Causes blurred vision and focusing difficulty; Glaucoma treatment

8. Adverse effects of acetylcholine include low _____ after system absorption, transient hypotension, decreased HR, bronchospasm, flushing and sweating

10. AKA Diamox; Used to treat glaucoma

12. AKA Carbonic anhydrase inhibitors

15. AKA Timolol

17. Miotic eye medications cause _____ of the pupil (of the eye) and ciliary muscle

18. AKA Isopto Eserine

19. AKA Phospholine Iodine; Clients must wash hands before use

20. Beoptic and Timoptic

Down

2. AKA Echothiophate

5. AKA Isopto Carpine

7. Treatment for glaucoma is _____; It should never be discontinued

9. AKA Physostigmine

10. AKA Miochol; Used to decrease intraocular pressure in glaucoma; Used to achieve miosis in cataract surgery

11. AKA Carbachol

13. AKA Trusopt; Used to treat glaucoma

14. AKA Acetazolamide; Classified as CAI

16. AKA Isopto Carbachol; Used for symptoms of eye and brow pain, photophobia, and blurred vision

Miotics

Dr. Evelyn J. Biluk

Word bank

ACETAZOLAMIDE   ACETYLCHOLINE   BETABLOCKERS   CAIS   CARBACHOL   CONTRACTION

DIAMOX   DORZOLAMIDE   ECHOTHIOPHATE   ISOPTOCARBACHOL   ISOPTOCARPINE

ISOPTOESERINE   LIFELONG   MIOCHOL   PHOSPHOLINEIODINE   PHYSOSTIGMINE   PILOCAR

PILOCARPINE   TIMOPTIC   TOXICITY   TRUSOPT

Miotics

Dr. Evelyn J. Biluk

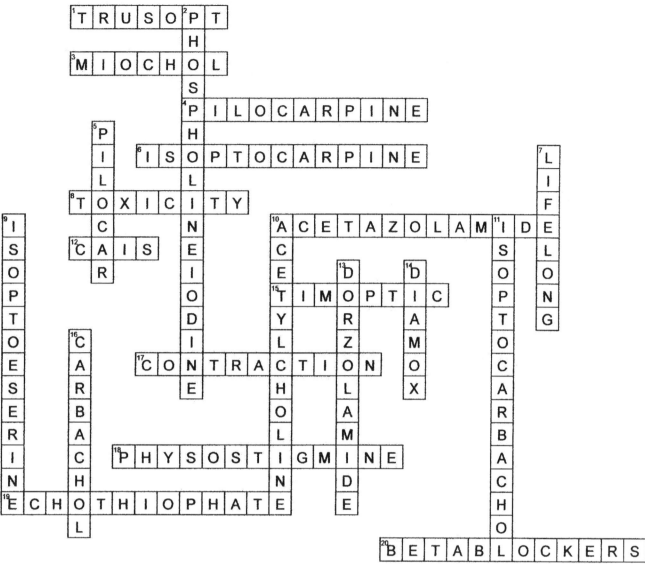

Cardiac Glycosides
Dr. Evelyn J. Biluk

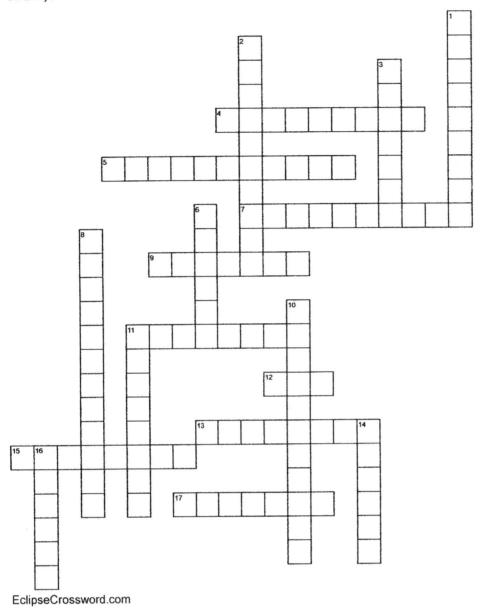

Cardiac Glycosides

Dr. Evelyn J. Biluk

Across

4. _____ - digoxin reaction may occur

5. Digoxin is used for paroxysmal atrial _____

7. AKA Inocor; Used for short-term management of CHF

9. Digoxin is eliminated by the _____

11. AKA Milrinone; Phosphodiesterase inhibitor

12. Lanoxin is used for congestive heart failure (_____)

13. _____ chronotropic effect involves decreasing the conduction rate

15. Digoxin antidote

17. AKA Lanoxin; Increased the force of myocardial contraction and decreases the rate of conduction while increasing the refractory period at the AV node

Down

1. AKA Primacor; Used for short-term management of CHF

2. Adverse effects of digoxin are _____ with a narrow margin of safety

3. AKA Digoxin

6. Avoid high-_____ foods while on digoxin

8. Lanoxin is used for atrial _____ and atrial flutter

10. Adverse effects of lanoxin include _____, anorexia, nausea, vomiting, diarrhea, headaches, fatigue, confusion, insomnia, convulsions, visual disturbances, blurred vision, green or yellow tint or halos and hypersensitivity

11. _____ inotropic effect improves blood supply to the vital organs and kidneys

14. Digoxin _____ is better absorbed by the GI tract

16. AKA Inamrinone

Cardiac Glycosides

Dr. Evelyn J. Biluk

Word bank

ARRHYTHMIAS   CHF   CUMULATIVE   DIGIBIND   DIGOXIN   ELIXIR   FIBRILLATION   INAMRINONE

INOCOR   KIDNEYS   LANOXIN   MILRINONE   NEGATIVE   POSITIVE   PRIMACOR   QUINIDINE

SODIUM   TACHYCARDIA

Cardiac Glycosides
Dr. Evelyn J. Biluk

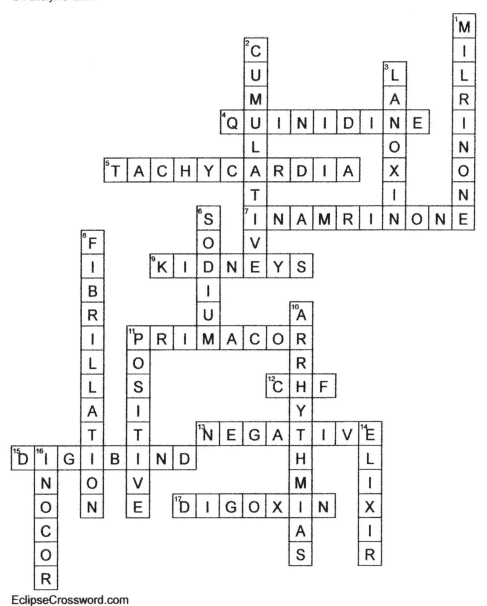

Antiarrhythmic Drugs

Dr. Evelyn J. Biluk

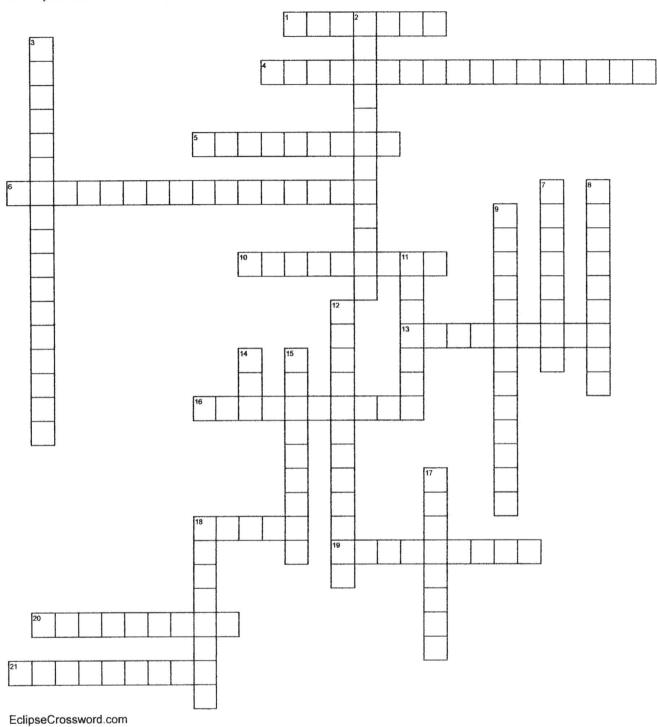

Antiarrhythmic Drugs

Dr. Evelyn J. Biluk

Across

1. AKA Calan

4. Adverse effect of digitalis

5. AKA Calan or Isoptin; Calcium channel blocker; Used for the management of chronic, stable *angina and the treatment of supraventricular* tachyrhythmias

6. Adverse effect of quinidine

10. Depresses myocardial excitability; Used in atrial fibrillation as well as flutter ventricular tachycardia

13. AKA Procainamide

16. AKA Procardia; Calcium channel blocker; Used in the management of chronic, stable angina and the treatment of supraventricular tachyrhythmias

18. AKA Isoptin

19. AKA Cardizem; Calcium channel blocker; Used in the management of chronic, stable angina and treatment of supraventricular tachyrhythmias

20. AKA Nifedipine

21. AKA Lidocaine

Down

2. AKA Pronestyl; Used to treat PVCs, ventricular tachycardia and some atrial arrhythmias

3. Adverse effect of pronestyl

7. Adverse effect of norpace

8. Used in treatment of CHF, atrial fibrillation and atrial flutter

9. Adverse effect of xylocaine

11. AKA Disopyramide

12. AKA Norpace; Used for PVCs and episodes of ventricular trachycardia; Increases action potential duration and effective refractory period of the atria and ventricles which decreases automaticity and conduction velocity

14. Patients on calcium channel blockers coupled with a beta blocker may develop _____

15. AKA Xylocaine; Used for acute ventricular arrhythmias

17. Adverse effect of digitalis

18. AKA Diltiazem

Antiarrhythmic Drugs

Dr. Evelyn J. Biluk

Word bank

CALAN   CARDIZEM   CHF   DIGITALIS   DILTIAZEM   DISOPYRAMIDE   DRYMOUTH   ISOPTIN

LIDOCAINE   NIFEDIPINE   NORPACE   PROCAINAMIDE   PROCARDIA   PRONESTYL   QUINIDINE

SEVEREHYPOTENSION   SLURREDSPEECH   THROMBOCYTOPENIA   TOXICITY   VERAPAMIL

XYLOCAINE   YELLOW-GREENHALOS

Antiarrhythmic Drugs

Dr. Evelyn J. Biluk

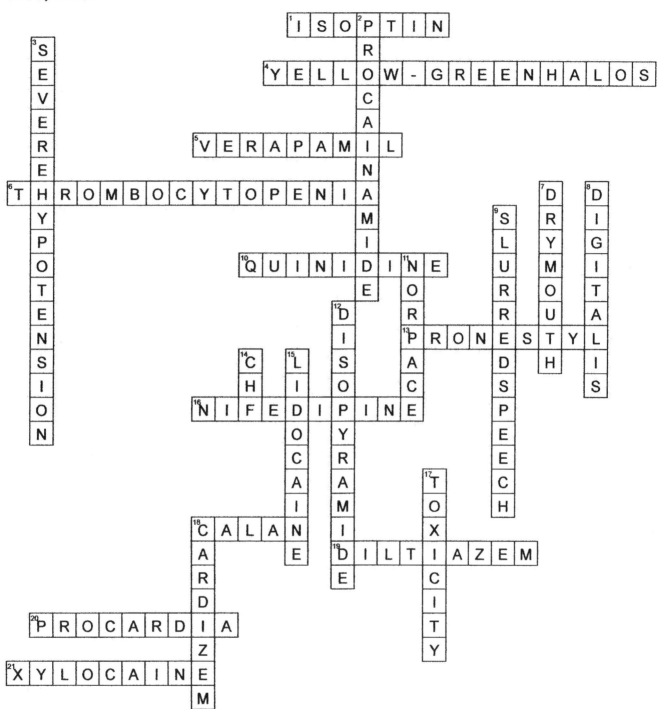

EclipseCrossword.com

Antianginal Drugs

Dr. Evelyn J. Biluk

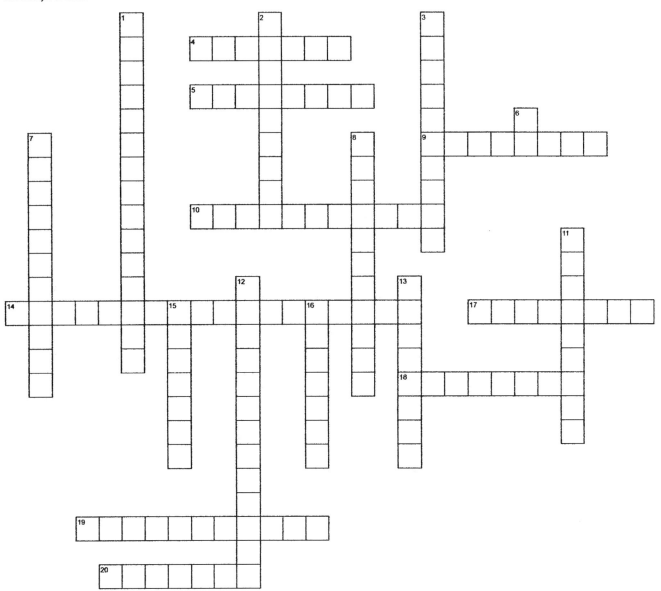

Antianginal Drugs

Dr. Evelyn J. Biluk

Across

4. _____ or acetaminophen can be given to patients for headache relief

5. Nitroglycerin should be taken before _____ to prevent an anginal attack

9. AKA Nitroglycerin

10. Verapamil can cause _____; Clients should take radial pulse before taking medication

14. AKA Isordil; Used to treat or prevent anginal attacks

17. Isordil can be given PO in _____ tablets

18. The back of a transdermal nitroglycerin patch contains _____

19. _____ patch can cause burns to clients standing near microwave ovens or if defibrillation is required

20. Calcium channel blocker; AKA Verapamil

Down

1. Used to manage CHF with acute MI; Also controls intraoperative hypotension or manages hypertension

2. AKA Nitroglycerin

3. Nitroglycerin given in this form at the onset of an attack or anticipation of an attack; 0.15 - 0.6 mg

6. Nitroglycerin given in this form as sustained release; 2.5 - 2.6 mg TID

7. _____ can occur in patients taking nitroglycerin and verapamil

8. AKA Nitroglycerin

11. AKA Calan or Isoptin; Used for angina, essential hypertension (PO form only) and cardiac dysrhythmias (IV use only)

12. Used to treat angina pectoris

13. _____ associated with nitroglycerin will discontinue with long-term use

15. AKA Isosorbide Dinitrate

16. _____ ointment is associated with skin rash

Antianginal Drugs

Dr. Evelyn J. Biluk

Word bank

ALUMINUM   ASPIRIN   BRADYCARDIA   CHEWABLE   EXERCISE   HEADACHE   HYPOTENSION

ISOPTIN   ISORDIL   ISOSORBIDDINITRATE   IVNITROGLYCERIN   NITRO-BID   NITRODUR

NITROGLYCERIN   NITROSTATIV   PO   SUBLINGUAL   TOPICAL   TRANSDERMAL   VERAPAMIL

Antianginal Drugs

Dr. Evelyn J. Biluk

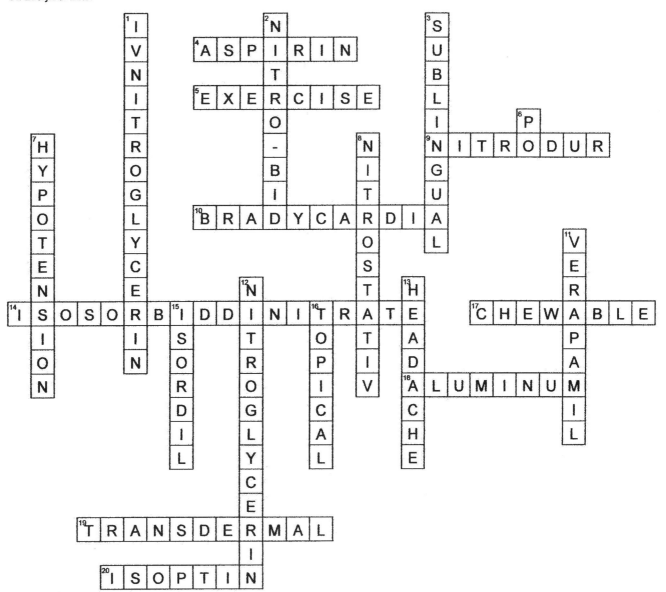

Peripheral Vasodilators and Antidysrhythmics I

Dr. Evelyn J. Biluk

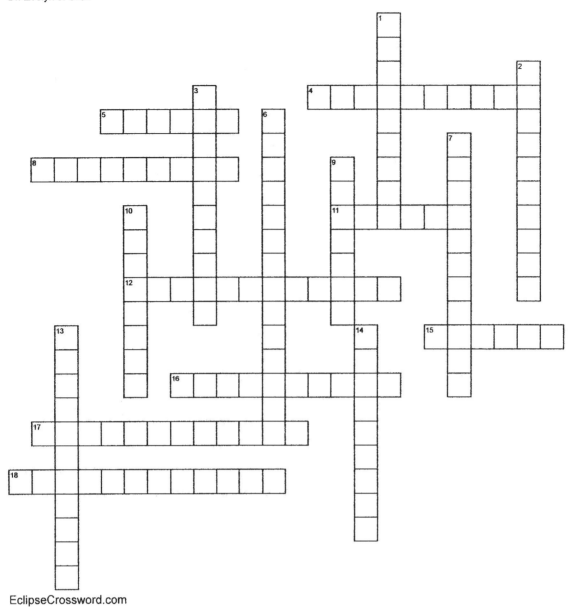

Peripheral Vasodilators and Antidysrhythmics I

Dr. Evelyn J. Biluk

Across

4. AKA Quinidine; Used for atrial dysrhythmias, atrial fibrillation and atrial flutter as well as ventricular dysrhythmias

5. AKA Chlopidogrel; Antiplatelet agent

8. Adverse effects of vasodilane can be dealt with by _____ of the dose

11. AKA Cilostazol; Antiplatelet agent

12. AKA Norpace; Used to treat PVCs and episodes of ventricular tachycardia

15. AKA Teclopidine; Antiplatelet agent

16. Adverse effects of antidysrhythmics include _____, GI distress, tinnitus, visual disturbances, dizziness, headahce, AV block, hypotension, thrombocytopenia, hypersensitivity, nausea, vomiting and diarrhea

17. AKA Persantine; Used to prevent thromboembolism and thromboembolic disorders

18. AKA Pronestyl; Used to treat PVCs, ventricular tachycardia and some atrial arrhythmias

Down

1. AKA Quinaglute

2. AKA Dipyridamole

3. AKA Pletal; Antiplatelet agent

6. AKA Vasodilan; Used to treat peripheral vascular disorders

7. AKA Ticlid; Antiplatelet agent

9. Commonly used antiplatelet agent; Available OTC

10. Adverse effects of peripheral vasodilators include _____, weakness, hypotension, GI distress, flushing and skin rashes

13. AKA Plavix; Antiplatelet agent

14. AKA Isoxsuprine HCl

Peripheral Vasodilators and Antidysrhythmics I

Dr. Evelyn J. Biluk

Word bank

ASPIRIN   CILOSTAZOL   CINCHONISM   CLOPIDOGREL   DIPYRIDAMOLE   DISOPYRAMIDE

HEADACHE   ISOXSUPRINEHCL   PERSANTINE   PLAVIX   PLETAL   PROCAINAMIDE   QUINAGLUTE

QUINIDINE   REDUCTION   TECLOPIDINE   TICLID   VASODILAN

Peripheral Vasodilators and Antidysrhythmics I

Dr. Evelyn J. Biluk

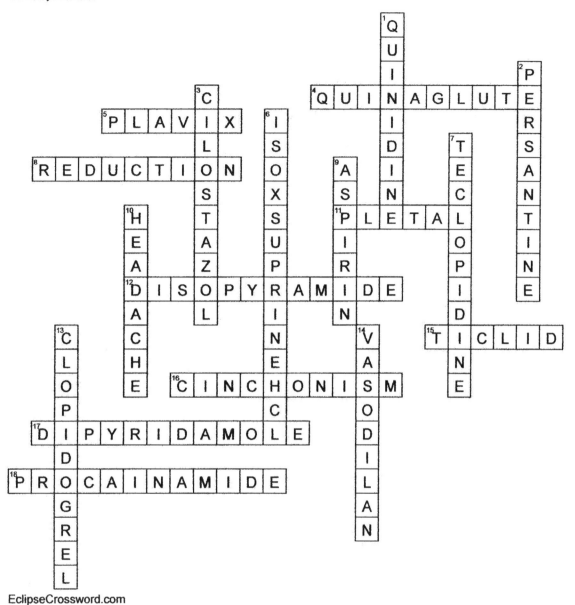

EclipseCrossword.com

Antidysrhythmics II

Dr. Evelyn J. Biluk

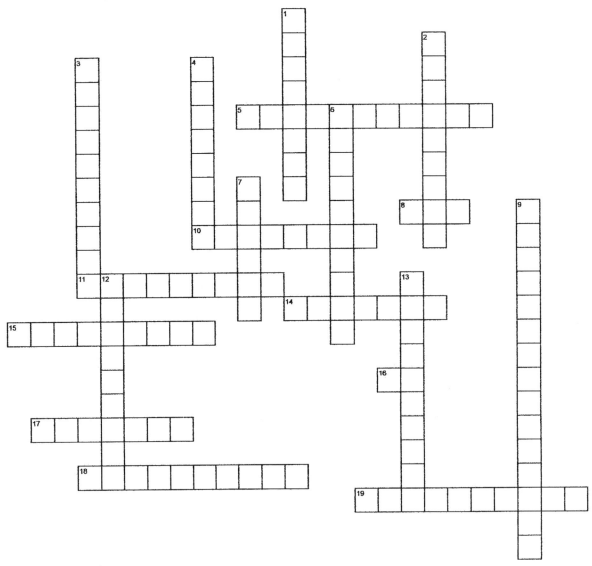

Antidysrhythmics II

Dr. Evelyn J. Biluk

Across

5. AKA Rythmol; Used to treat ventricular dysrhythmias

8. Adverse effects of xylocaine include _____ stimulation leading to seizures

10. AKA Phenytoin Sodium

11. AKA Moricizine

14. AKA Propafenone

15. AKA Xylocaine; Used for ventricular arrhythmias and as a local anesthetic

16. Xylocaine, tambocor and rythmol are all Class _____ drugs

17. AKA mexiletine

18. Adverse effects of lidocaine include _____, hypertension, bradycardia, ventricular tachycardia, drowsiness and CNS stimulation (leading to seizures)

19. AKA Tambocor; Used to treat ventricular dysrhythmias

Down

1. AKA Flecainide

2. AKA Lidocaine

3. AKA Mexitel

4. AKA Tocainide

6. Dilantin has high _____ and can precipitate easily

7. 0.9 % normal _____ is used to flush IV line and site to minimize venous irritation and prevent precipitation caused by phenytoin sodium

9. AKA Dilantin

12. AKA Tonocard

13. AKA Ethmozine; Used to treat life-threatening ventricular dysrhythmias; Sodium channel blocker

Antidysrhythmics II

Dr. Evelyn J. Biluk

Word bank

1C   ALKALINITY   CNS   DILANTIN   ETHMOZINE   FLECAINIDE   HEARTBLOCK   LIDOCAINE

MEXILETINE   MEXITEL   MORICIZINE   PHENYTOINSODIUM   PROPAFENONE   RYTHMOL   SALINE

TAMBOCOR   TOCAINIDE   TONOCARD   XYLOCAINE

Antidysrhythmics II

Dr. Evelyn J. Biluk

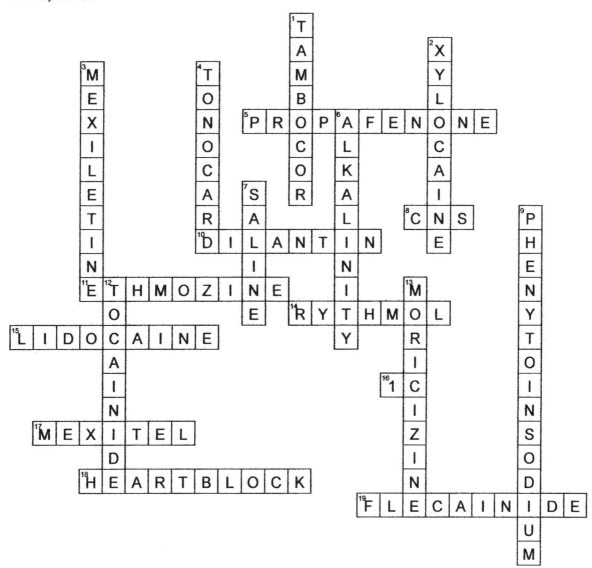

Beta Blockers

Dr. Evelyn J. Biluk

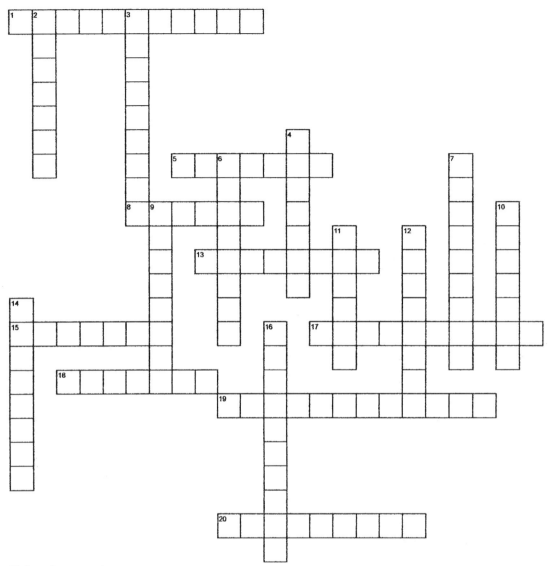

Beta Blockers

Dr. Evelyn J. Biluk

Across

1. Inderal is classified as a _____

5. AKA Corgard; Used to treat essential hypertension and angina

8. This pulse is taken before administering inderal

13. AKA Atenolol

15. AKA Propranolol

17. AKA Lopressor; Classified as a Class II antidysrhythmic; Given after an MI to decrease the risk of sudden cardiac death; Used to treat angina and hypertension

18. AKA Betapase; Classified as a Class III antidysrhythmic; Used to treat life-threatening ventricular dysrhythmias (such as ventricular tachycardia)

19. Adverse effects of inderal include _____, dizziness, drowsiness, insomnia, depression, bronchospasm, bradycardia, heart block, hypotension and rash

20. AKA Timolol

Down

2. AKA Brevibloc; Classified as Class II antidysrhythmic; Used to treat tachycardia, supraventricular tachycardia, atrial fibrillation and atrial flutter

3. AKA Metoprolol

4. AKA Nadolol

6. If a client is taking inderal and _____, he/she is more prone to developing hypoglycemia

7. AKA Esmolol

9. AKA Tenormin; Classified as a Class II antidysrhythmic; Used to treat angina and hypertension

10. AKA Blocadren; Used to treat essential hypertension

11. AKA Pindolol

12. AKA Sotalol

14. AKA Visken; Used to treat essential hypertension

16. AKA Inderal; Used to treat cardiac arrhythmias caused by excessive cardiac stimulation of sympathetic nerve impulse, digitalis-induced arrhythmias, essential hypertension, angina pectoris, preoperative management of pheochromocytoma and prevention of migraine headaches

Beta Blockers

Dr. Evelyn J. Biluk

Word bank

ATENOLOL   BETABLOCKER   BETAPASE   BLOCADREN   BREVIBLOC   CORGARD   DIABETIC

ESMOLOL   HYPOGLYCEMIA   INDERAL   LOPRESSOR   METOPROLOL   NADOLOL   PINDOLOL

PROPANOLOL   RADIAL   SOTALOL   TENORMIN   TIMOLOL   VISKEN

Beta Blockers

Dr. Evelyn J. Biluk

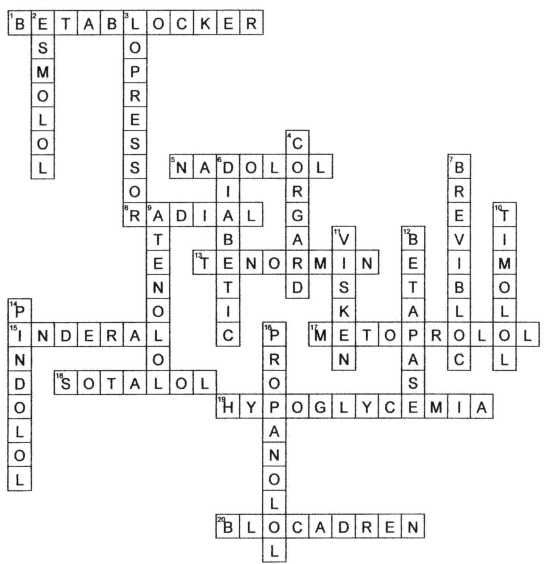

Cardiac Stimulants

Dr. Evelyn J. Biluk

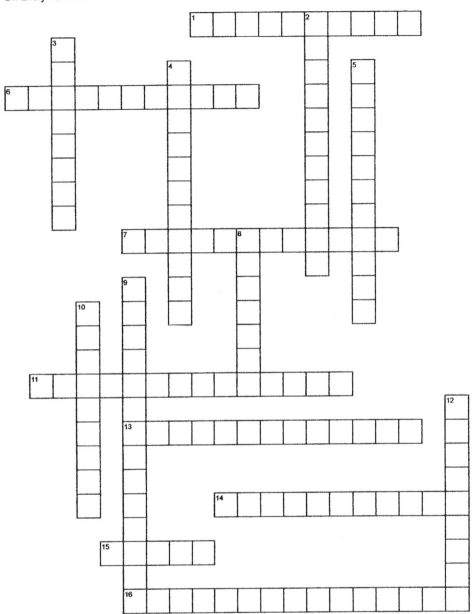

Cardiac Stimulants

Dr. Evelyn J. Biluk

Across

1. Isuprel is used to treat cardiac _____

6. Atropine sulfate acts systematically to block _____ activity throughout the human body

7. Isuprel is used to treat _____ hypersensitivity

11. Isuprel is also a _____

13. AKA Isuprel

14. _____ syndrome is treated with isoproteronol

15. Isuprel stimulates _____ adrenergic receptors in the heart

16. _____ blocks vagal stimulation of the SA node in the heart resulting in an increased HR

Down

2. Atropine sulfate is also used to manage _____ sinus bradycardia

3. Adverse effects of atropine sulfate are related to the _____ of cholinergic activity in the human body

4. Atropine sulfate is used to treat sinus _____ or asystole

5. _____ arrhythmias are treated using isuprel

8. AKA Isoproteronol

9. Adverse effects of isuprel include _____, headache, palpitations, dry mouth, flushing and sweating

10. Cardiac stimulants are _____ nervous system drugs

12. Atropine sulfate is also used to diagnose _____ dysfunction

Cardiac Stimulants

Dr. Evelyn J. Biluk

Word bank

ATROPINESULFATE   AUTONOMIC   BETA1   BLOCKING   BRADYCARDIA   BRONCHIALEDEMA

BRONCHODILATOR   CAROTIDSINUS   CHOLINERGIC   ISOPROTERONOL   ISUPREL   SINUSNODE

STANDSTILL   STOKESADAMS   SYMPTOMATIC   VENTRICULAR

Cardiac Stimulants

Dr. Evelyn J. Biluk

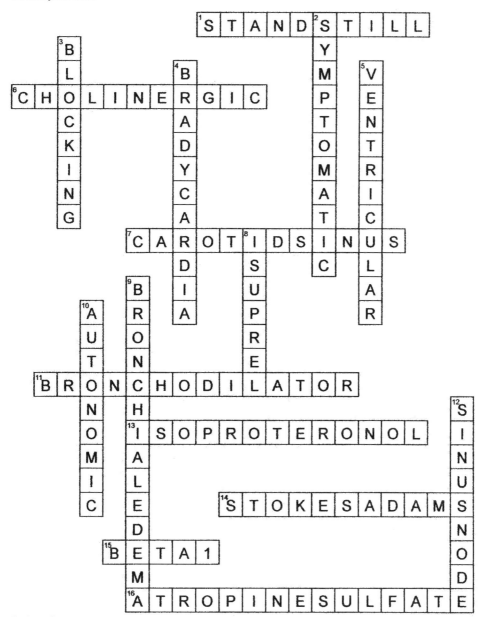

Anticoagulants
Dr. Evelyn J. Biluk

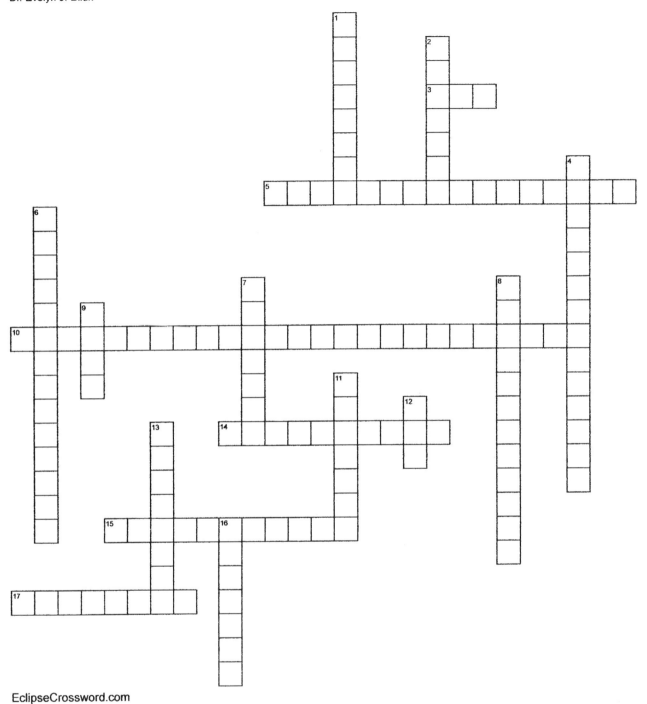

Anticoagulants

Dr. Evelyn J. Biluk

Across

3. AKA Partial Thromboplastin Time

5. _____ is an antidote for heparin overdose

10. AKA LMWH; Removes part of the heparin molecules resulting in a smaller, more accurate heparin; Used for DVT and PE especially after hip/knee or abdominal surgery

14. AKA Lovenox

15. Anticoagulants inhibit at least one of the steps involved in the _____ process

17. Adverse effects of LMWH include _____, anemia and thrombocytopenia

Down

1. Continuous IV infusion of heparin requires _____ monitoring to ensure accuracy in dose

2. _____ blocks the conversion of prothrombin to thrombin as well as fibrinogen to fibrin

4. AKA Coumadin; Blocks prothrombin synthesis

6. _____ do not dissolve existing blood clots but prevent further coagulation from happening

7. AKA Dalteprin

8. Changing the dose of coumadin by missing a dose on one day and then doubling the dose on the next day is _____ and will negatively affect the blood coagulation

9. AKA Low Molecular Weight Heparin

11. A patient on heparin should not take _____ due to increased risk of bleeding

12. _____ (disseminated intravascular clotting syndrome) is treated using heparin

13. AKA Warfarin Sodium

16. AKA Enoxaparin

Anticoagulants

Dr. Evelyn J. Biluk

Word bank

ANTICOAGULANTS   ASPIRIN   BLEEDING   COAGULATION   CONSTANT   COUMADIN   DIC
ENOXAPARIN   FRAGMIN   HEPARIN   LMWH   LOVENOX   LOWMOLECULARWEIGHTHEPARIN
PROTAMINESULFATE   PTT   UNACCEPTABLE   WARFARINSODIUM

Anticoagulants

Dr. Evelyn J. Biluk

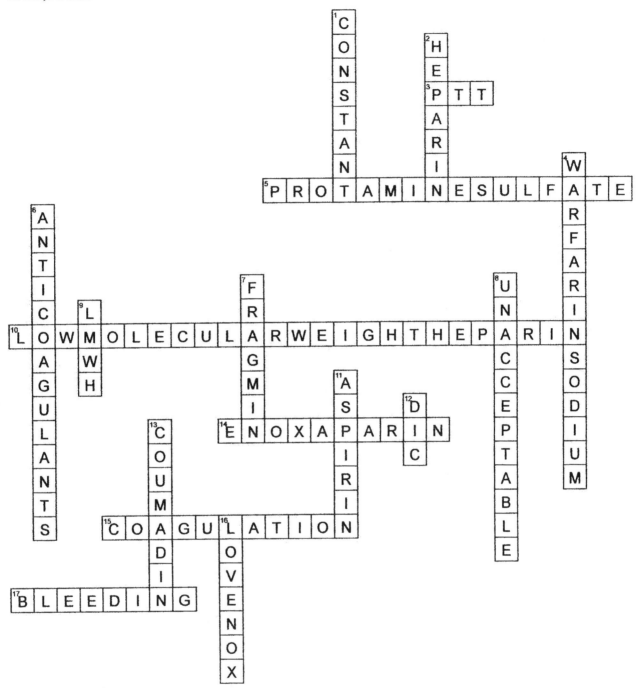

Thrombolytic Drugs

Dr. Evelyn J. Biluk

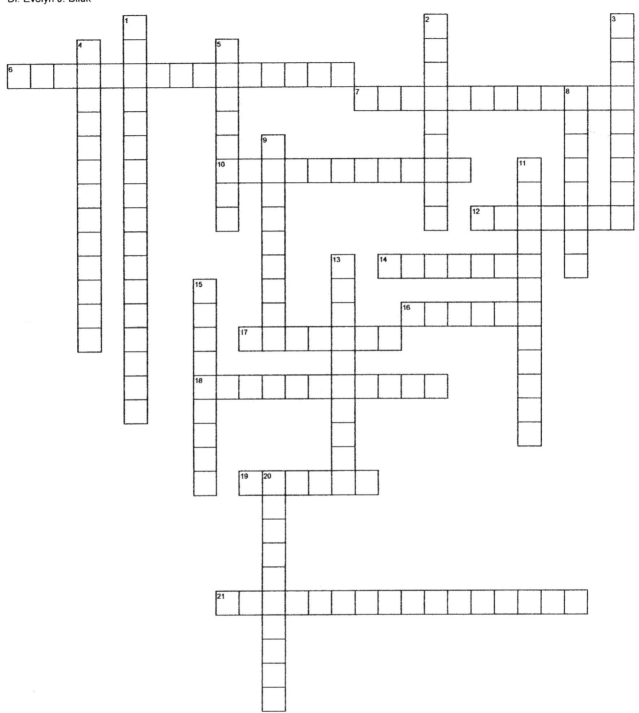

Thrombolytic Drugs

Dr. Evelyn J. Biluk

Across

6. _____ are given to clients in order to decrease allergic reaction to streptase

7. AKA TNKase

10. Adverse effects of streptokinase include _____, bleeding and allergic reaction

12. AKA Anistreplase

14. _____ is needed when a client is receiving streptase

16. AKA Tenecteplase

17. _____ must be discontinued before a client is started on streptokinase

18. Streptase transforms _____ into plasmin

19. Streptokinase is normally reconstituted with normal _____ or 5 % dextrose solution

21. _____ is the antidote for streptokinase

Down

1. The client needs to be monitored for _____ every 15 minutes for the first treatment hour, every 30 minutes for the second through eighth hours, and then every 8 hours

2. AKA Activase

3. AKA Streptokinase; Used for pulmonary emboli, coronary artery thrombosis, deep venous thrombosis, and arteriovenous cannula occlusion

4. AKA Streptase

5. AKA Reteplase

8. AKA Alteplase

9. AKA Abbokinase

11. AKA Eminase

13. Plasmin degrades _____, fibrin clots and other plasma proteins

15. AKA Retavase

20. AKA Urokinase

Thrombolytic Drugs

Dr. Evelyn J. Biluk

Word bank

ABBOKINASE   ACTIVASE   ALTEPLASE   AMINOCAPROICACID   ANISTREPLASE   ARRHYTHMIAS

BEDREST   CORTICOSTEROIDS   EMINASE   EXCESSIVEBLEEDING   FIBRINOGEN   HEPARIN

PLASMINOGEN   RETAVASE   RETEPLASE   SALINE   STREPTASE   STREPTOKINASE   TENECTEPLASE

TNKASE   UROKINASE

Thrombolytic Drugs

Dr. Evelyn J. Biluk

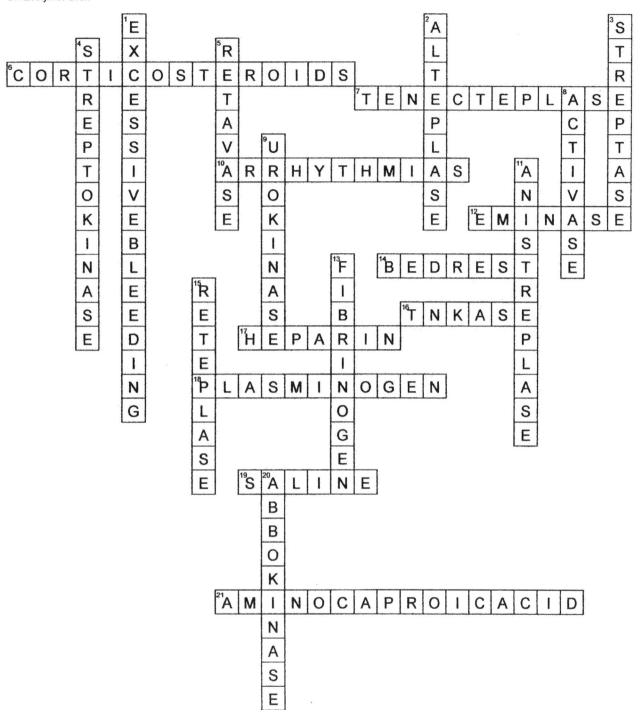

Antilipemic Agents

Dr. Evelyn J. Biluk

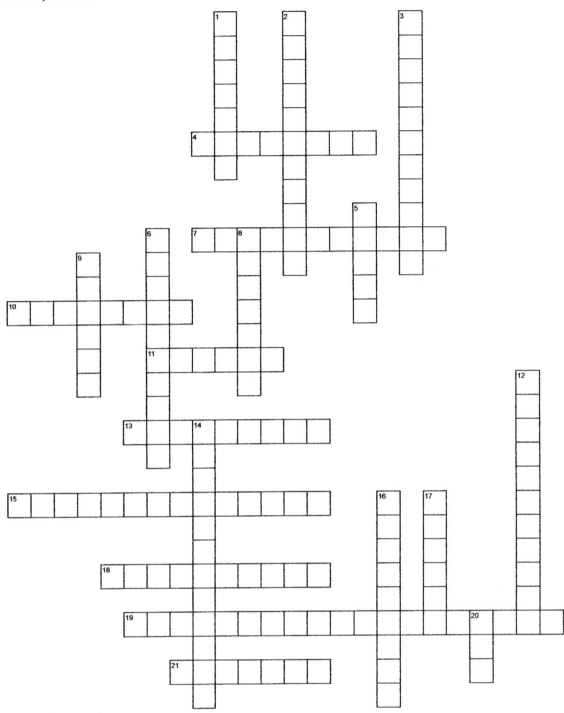

Antilipemic Agents

Dr. Evelyn J. Biluk

Across

4. AKA Colestipol

7. AKA Lopid; Decreases triglycerides and increases HDL cholesterol

10. AKA Cholestyramine

11. AKA Fenofibrate

13. AKA Nicobid or Niacin; Reduces liver synthesis and reduces cholesterol and total lipid levels

15. AKA Questran; Used to treat Type IIa hyperlipoproteinemia and pruritus (caused by partial biliary obstruction)

18. AKA Colestid; Similar in action to questran

19. Adverse effects of questran include _____ of A, D and K as well as as constipation, nausea, vomiting, rash, skin irritation, osteoporosis, headache, dizziness, syncope, arthritis and fever

21. AKA Vitamin B3

Down

1. AKA Atorvastatin

2. AKA Pravachol; Classified as a reductase inhibitor; Decreases cholesterol levels

3. AKA Lescol; Classified as a reductase inhibitor; Decreases cholesterol levels

5. AKA Gemfibrozil

6. AKA Mevacor; Classified as a reductase inhibitor; Decreases cholesterol levels

8. AKA Lovastatin

9. AKA Fluvastatin

12. AKA Tricor; Decrease triglycerides and increases HDL cholesterol

14. AKA Lipitor; Classified as reductase inhibitor; Decreases cholesterol levels

16. AKA Pravastatin

17. Cholestyramine should be taken _____ meals for improved absorption

20. Adverse effects of lipitor, lescol, mevacor and pravachol include elevated _____, headache, insomnia, fatigue, blurred vision, myalgias, nausea, hepatotoxicity, and elevated alkaline phosphatase and transaminase levels

Antilipemic Agents

Dr. Evelyn J. Biluk

Word bank

ATORVASTATIN   BEFORE   CHOLESTYRAMINE   COLESTID   COLESTIPOL   CPK   FENOFIBRATE

FLUVASTATIN   GEMFIBROZIL   LESCOL   LIPITOR   LOPID   LOVASTATIN   MEVACOR   NICOBID

PRAVACHOL   PRAVASTATIN   QUESTRAN   TRICOR   VITAMINB3   VITAMINDEFICIENCIES

Antilipemic Agents

Dr. Evelyn J. Biluk

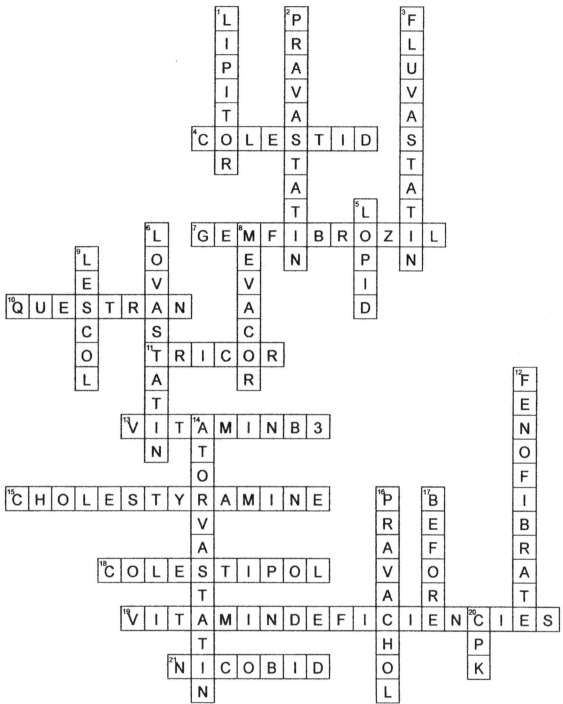

EclipseCrossword.com

Antihypertensives I

Dr. Evelyn J. Biluk

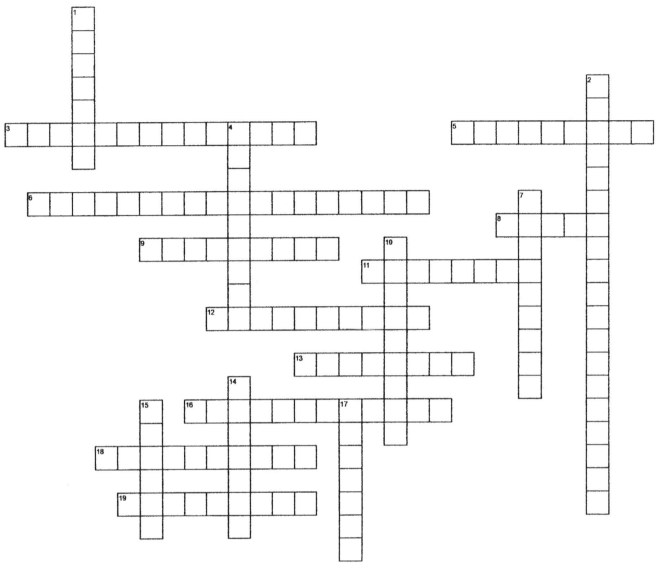

Antihypertensives I

Dr. Evelyn J. Biluk

Across

3. Serpalan lowers BP by blocking _____ in CNS and peripherally

5. AKA Cardura

6. Adverse effects of serpalan include _____, drowsiness, nasal obstruction, impotence, decreased cardiac output, postural hypotension, diarrhea, increased gastric secretions

8. Minipress is classified as an _____ adrenergic receptor blocker

9. AKA Clonidine

11. AKA Reserpine

12. Serpalan is a _____ -acting adrenergic neuron blocker

13. AKA Minipress; Used for essential hypertension and hypertension caused by pheochromocytoma

16. AKA Ismelin; Rarely used

18. AKA Aldomet; May cause blood dyscrasias and hepatotoxicity

19. AKA Prazosin

Down

1. AKA Methyldopa

2. Adverse effects of minipress include _____ and syncope with initial therapy

4. AKA Serpalan; Rarely used

7. AKA Catapress; Used alone or in combo with other antihypertensives

10. AKA Hytrin

14. AKA Doxazosin

15. AKA Terazosin

17. AKA Guanethidine

Antihypertensives I

Dr. Evelyn J. Biluk

Word bank

ALDOMET   ALPHA   CARDURA   CATAPRESS   CLONIDINE   DOXAZOSIN   GUANETHIDINE   HYTRIN

ISMELIN   METHYLDOPA   MINIPRESS   NOREPINEPHRINE   PERIPHERAL   POSTURALHYPOTENSION

PRAZOSIN   RESERPINE   SERPALAN   SUICIDALDEPRESSION   TERAZOSIN

Antihypertensives I

Dr. Evelyn J. Biluk

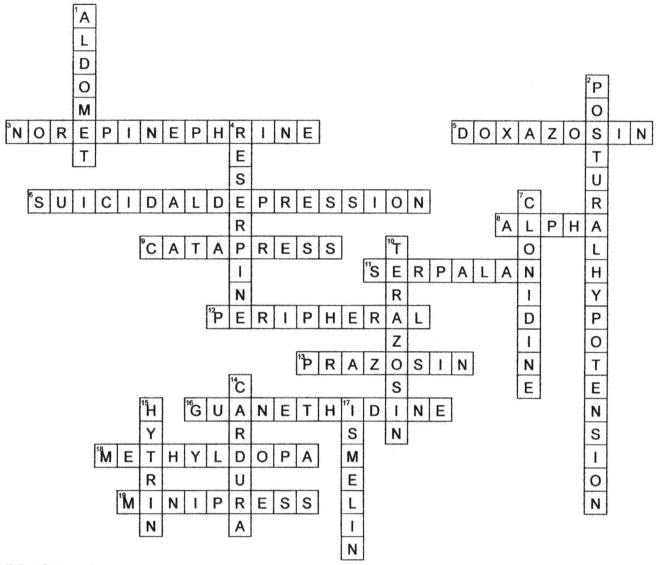

Antihypertensives II

Dr. Evelyn J. Biluk

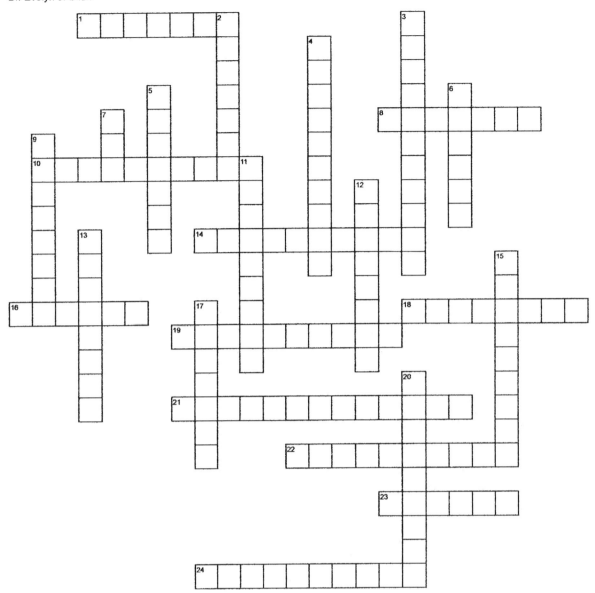

Antihypertensives II

Dr. Evelyn J. Biluk

Across

1. AKA Lisinopril

8. AKA Captopril

10. AKA Hydralazine

14. AKA Diovan

16. AKA Ramipril

18. AKA Fosinopril

19. AKA Zestril

21. AKA Nipride; Used to treat hypertensive emergencies; Given as an IV

22. AKA Monopril

23. AKA Valasartan

24. AKA Lotensin

Down

2. AKA Minoxidil

3. AKA Apresoline; Classified as a direct-acting vasodilator

4. Adverse effects of ACE inhibitors includes blood _____, hypotension, proteinuria, hyperkalemia, rash and loss of taste perception

5. AKA Enalapril

6. AKA Losarten

7. Captopril is an _____ inhibitor

9. AKA Altace

11. AKA Vasotec

12. AKA Benezepril

13. AKA Cozaar

15. AKA Capoten; Used to treat essential hypertension (with normal renal function), severe hypertension (with renal dysfunction) and CHF

17. AKA Nitroprusside

20. AKA Loniten; Topical preparation is called Rogaine

Antihypertensives II

Dr. Evelyn J. Biluk

Word bank

ACE   ALTACE   APRESOLINE   BENEZEPRIL   CAPOTEN   CAPTOPRIL   COZAAR   DIOVAN

DYSCRASIAS   ENALAPRIL   FOSINOPRIL   HYDRAZALINE   LISINOPRIL   LONITEN   LOSARTEN

LOTENSIN   MINOXIDIL   MONOPRIL   NIPRIDE   NITROPRUSSIDE   RAMIPRIL   VALASARTAN

VASOTEC   ZESTRIL

Antihypertensives II

Dr. Evelyn J. Biluk

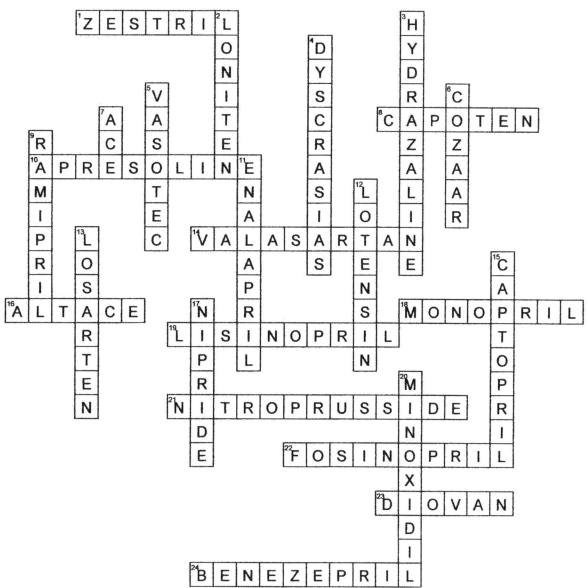

35345916R00131

Made in the USA
Lexington, KY
07 September 2014